Understanding BPPV

Outlining the causes and effects of Benign Paroxysmal Positional Vertigo

Mark Knoblauch, PhD

KP Kiremma Press

Disclaimer: This book is not intended as a substitute for the medical advice of licensed physicians. The reader should regularly consult a physician in matters relating to his/her health and particularly with respect to any symptoms that may require diagnosis or medical attention.

For more of Mark's books, please visit his website at www.authorMK.com

ISBN: 978-1-7320674-1-7

This book is simply dedicated to everyone that has had to deal with the at-first frightening, then annoying symptoms of BPPV.

Contents

Introduction

Benign paroxysmal positional vertigo. *BPPV.* One might wonder if any other medical condition's name is more intimidating or takes more effort to say. If you're reading this book, there's a strong likelihood that you either have previously or are currently dealing with the distinct displeasure of the effects of BPPV. Rest assured that you are not alone. As we will discuss in this book, BPPV is one of the most common vertigo-associated conditions. Perhaps more important for you to understand is that true BPPV – despite its sometimes forceful symptoms – is relatively harmless in nature and typically amounts to nothing more than an annoyance.

Let me be clear – I say 'true BPPV' is relatively harmless because it is imperative that you have actually been diagnosed by a medical professional with BPPV, and are not instead relying on a self-diagnosis based upon something you might have heard from a friend or read on the internet. Other medical conditions can mimic the symptoms of BPPV but are in many cases more serious and require a more intense intervention. Therefore, if you are experiencing vertigo-associated symptoms, even if only during certain head movements, it is essential that you undergo a thorough evaluation by a medical professional trained in vestibular disorders.

If you or someone you know has been diagnosed with BPPV, this book is designed to help provide you information necessary to help you better understand BPPV both as a medical condition and how it can affect your life. In writing this book it was my intent to include information I wish I had known when I was experiencing the effects of BPPV myself almost 20 years ago. Back then, our understanding of BPPV was relatively new, and as a result the research that we had available was somewhat limited. Since that time our insights into the factors involved with BPPV have grown tremendously, and it is my hope that this book has been written in a way that details this improved understanding of BPPV.

Therefore, we will first review the relevant ear anatomy, focusing specifically on those portions of the ear most involved with BPPV. The anatomy associated with our equilibrium system is quite extensive, and while the structure and function of the inner ear is quite intricate, I feel that it is important to point out those components specifically involved with BPPV. Next, we will look at just what BPPV is, combining what we learned in the anatomy chapter with the series of events that lead up to the symptoms of BPPV.

We will also look at the most serious form of BPPV, known as 'intractable BPPV' that does not respond to traditional treatment of BPPV. While intractable BPPV has the same cause as traditional BPPV, the symptoms can be more severe – and the treatments less effective – than the more common forms of BPPV. Then, to outline my own experience with BPPV, I detail my time living with positional vertigo, including how it happened and how I was finally able to receive a diagnosis and treatment towards the frustrating and annoying bouts of positional vertigo.

We then look at the various diagnostic tests and treatments available for BPPV, with particular focus toward the various repositioning techniques used in successfully treating this condition. Despite a similarity in symptoms, there are actually many different variations of BPPV specific to the inner ear's structure, and I feel that it is important to outline the various techniques used in treating the multiple forms of BPPV. Then, we will review other inner ear conditions that can present vertigo-related symptoms similar to those of BPPV. Finally, we will look at the influence BPPV can have on an individual's quality of life.

If you or someone you know is experiencing the effects of BPPV, this book is intended to be a source of information that outlines for you what is going on within the structures of your inner ear, as well as what you can expect regarding the condition. Understand, however, that it is not designed to serve as a self-diagnosis or self-treatment guide. Instead, it is written to serve as a resource after your BPPV diagnosis in order to help you understand the underlying events occurring with BPPV.

I hope that you find this book informative, and that you benefit from the information contain within. After all, it was written for you, by someone who has been through what you are going through.

Mark Knoblauch

Chapter 1: Anatomy of the Ear

MOST OF US TEND TO THINK of our ear in terms of the part that we can see on the side of our head. However, the ear is much more than that. In fact, the *pinna* – the part of the ear that we can see – is actually the least involved structure of all. The truly functional parts of our ears exist deep inside of our skulls and are comprised of very delicate structures. Because of their delicate nature, the sensitive components of our inner ear are subject to damage due to causes such as trauma, such as might occur when getting hit in the head with a ball, or disease, as could occur due to a serious ear infection. Injury to the structures of the ear can cause not only diminished hearing or deafness, but also a variety of vestibular-related problems such as dizziness, unsteadiness, or vertigo.

Although we know that the inner ear is involved in hearing and equilibrium, it is important to understand that the ear merely *detects* sound and motion – it does not 'interpret' sound nor process any motion that we make. Rather, processing is a function of our brain that occurs in response to input received from sensors deep within our ear structure. Because the brain and portions of the inner ear work together to detect and process movement, the inner ear is often noted as the 'peripheral vestibular organ'.

As you are aware, BPPV is itself a condition of the ear. But rather than being the result of true 'damage' to the structures of the inner ear, BPPV involves more of a 'disruption' of ear structures. In order to orient you to the parts of the ear involved in BPPV, this chapter is designed to provide a general overview of ear anatomy along with a specific look at those structures thought to be directly involved in BPPV. While we will discuss the inner ear's role in hearing and balance, keep in mind that the anatomy and physiology of the inner ear involved with BPPV is related largely to those structures responsible for detecting motion, not actually interpreting motion.

Outer ear

The outer ear is the portion of the ear that we can see (Figure 1.1). This includes the large pinna as well as the ear canal that leads to the eardrum. The function of the outer ear is to funnel sound to the eardrum, and as it is located well away from the inner ear structures, the outer ear is not involved in BPPV.

Middle ear

The middle ear is the air-filled portion of the ear located behind the eardrum and housed within the temporal bone (Figure 1.1). This portion of the ear holds the three small bones – the malleus, stapes, and incus – that transfer sound from the eardrum to the inner ear. As with the outer ear, the middle ear is not involved specifically with BPPV.

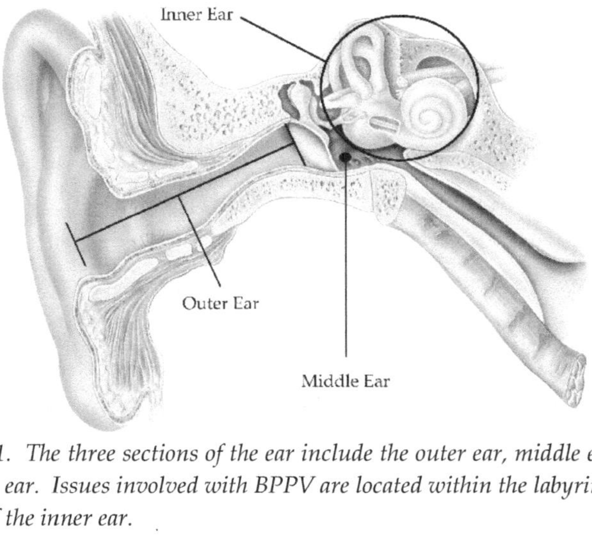

Figure 1.1. The three sections of the ear include the outer ear, middle ear, and inner ear. Issues involved with BPPV are located within the labyrinth portion of the inner ear.

Inner ear

The inner ear is the portion of the ear responsible for both conversion of sound waves to neural impulses as well as the perception and interpretation of body positioning. The inner ear is comprised of highly sensitive structures, which in turn makes the inner ear susceptible to injury. Because of the high level of involvement of the inner ear structures, the inner ear is one of the most intensively studied areas of vertebrate anatomy and physiology[1]. Despite its small size, damage to the intricate components of the inner ear can affect hearing as well as equilibrium, and even minor disruptive events can trigger several symptoms such as motion sickness, vertigo or nausea.

There are two predominant components that make up the inner ear – the cochlea and the vestibular system. Together, these two structures make up what is known as the *labyrinth.* It should be noted that the labyrinth organs are not free-standing organs; rather, they are actually tunnels through the temporal bone. These tunnels contain membranes that serve to contain the fluid (i.e. 'endolymph') housed within the labyrinth (Figure 1.2).

Because both the cochlea and vestibular organs are housed within the temporal bone, any traumatic force such as a punch to the head can be transferred directly to these structures. As we will note later, trauma to the head is in fact one cause of BPPV, initiating approximately 15% of BPPV cases[2].

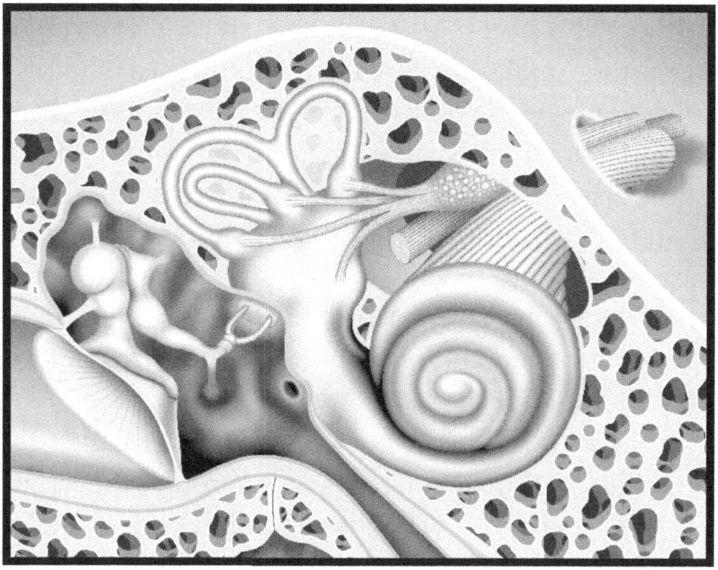

Figure 1.2. The cochlea and vestibular system are housed within the matrix of the temporal bone. Though actually formed by the bone, the labyrinth organs are lined with membranes that house the endolymph fluid of the inner ear.

Cochlea

The cochlea is a coiled, bony cavity resembling a snail shell within the temporal bone that is approximately three to four centimeters long[3] (Figure 1.3). Structurally, the cochlea has been described as being housed within the hardest bone matrix in the body[3]. The main function of the cochlea is to convert sound waves from the eardrum into nerve impulses, which are then sent to the brain for interpretation as sound. This occurs as a result of vibrations received from the small bones of the middle ear, known collectively as the ossicles. As the eardrum moves in response to sound waves, it transmits vibrations to the ossicles. One of the ossicles, known as the stirrup, is attached directly to the oval window membrane located on the cochlea. As this oval window membrane vibrates back and forth in response to the stirrup's movements, the vibrations are transmitted into the fluid-filled cochlea.

Inside of the cochlea is a structure called the organ of Corti that snakes its way through the length of the cochlea. The organ of Corti contains approximately 15,000 hair cells responsible for detecting vibrations within the cochlear fluid[4]. Higher-pitched sounds activate hair cells near the oval window while lower-pitched sounds stimulate hair cells further down the cochlea. Therefore, damage to a specific part of the cochlea can affect an individual's perception of that corresponding sound frequency. For example, damage to the cochlea near the oval window, where higher-pitched sounds are detected, would likely reduce an individual's ability to hear sounds such as a bell, or a bird chirping.

Vestibular system

The vestibular system of the inner ear serves to detect body motion as well as head position. It is now well-accepted that the structures making up the vestibular organs are involved in BPPV, so we will outline in detail the relevant anatomy of the vestibular organs.

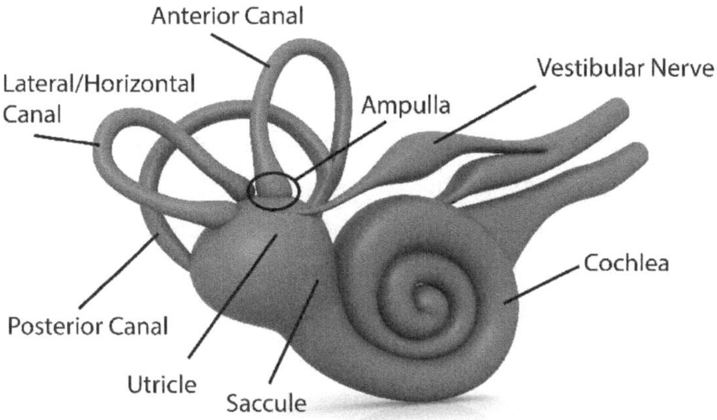

Figure 1.3. The labyrinth system is a specialized structure consisting of organs used for detection of sound as well as registering head motion.

Five independent structures are involved in our ability to detect motion. The first two structures are the saccule and the utricle, both of which contain small crystals that play a predominant role in detecting motion. Because they house these small crystals, known as otoliths, the utricle and saccule are known as the "otolith organs". The remainder of the vestibular organ is comprised of three 'tubes' called semicircular canals which form loops through the temporal bone. The utricle, saccule, and semicircular canals are largely responsible for the symptoms associated with BPPV, and as such we will look closely at the anatomy of each.

Saccule

The saccule is a bulged-out portion of the labyrinth responsible for detecting vertical motion of the head. For example, jumping up and down or riding in an elevator are activities that activate the motion sensors within the saccule. The saccule lies near the bottom of the vestibular structures, close to the entrance of the cochlea.

Within the saccule is a structure called the *macula sacculi,* a vertically-oriented organ which houses a two- to three-millimeter area comprised of sensory hair cells responsible for detecting head motion. The ends of these hair cells extend horizontally and are covered by a gelatinous layer, over which is a fibrous structure called the otolithic membrane. This otolithic membrane is embedded with thousands of crystals known by a variety of names including *statoconia, otoconia,* and *otolith.* For the purpose of this book we will use the term *otolith* to describe the crystals of the ear.

Because it is embedded with *otoliths,* the otolithic membrane is heavier than the structures around it. Therefore, when the body moves in a vertical plane such as occurs when jumping, gravity pulls the otoliths downward. This causes the hair cells to bend, which in turn sends a signal to the brain that is interpreted as vertical motion of the head.

Utricle

The utricle is larger than the saccule and serves to detect when the head moves in the horizontal plane. This would include forward, backward, or side-to-side motion of the head. Motions which activate the utricle include the sensation experienced when taking off in an airplane, or when riding in a car as it turns a corner. Like the saccule, the utricle contains a macula called the *macula utriculi.* In contrast to the saccule's vertically-oriented macula, the macula utriculi is positioned horizontally with hair cells that are positioned vertically. The mechanism by which the macula utriculi detects motion operates similarly to that of the macula saccule in that the hair cells are covered with a gelatinous layer which is in turn overlaid with an otolithic membrane embedded with otoliths.

When forward, backward, or side-to-side head motion occurs, the inertia created from the force of the motion upon the embedded otoliths creates a sort of 'shearing' motion between the gelatinous layer and the otolithic membrane. This motion is then detected by the utricle's hair cells which send a signal to the brain that is interpreted as the respective directional motion of the head.

Otoliths

Because of the otolith's involvement in BPPV it is relevant to provide a specific overview of what these small crystalline structures are. Otoliths are microscopic (approximately 0.0004 inches long), calcium carbonate structures of the inner ear. The chemical structure of otoliths – calcium carbonate – is effectively the same structure as limestone, thereby providing weight to the crystals.

As we have discussed, the otoliths are embedded within the otolithic membrane. At rest, the otolithic membrane is stationary and the body does not receive any significant signal from the hair cells located in the layer underneath the otolithic membrane. When the head moves, however, the motion causes the otolithic membrane to lag slightly behind due to the accumulated weight of the otoliths. The brain senses this slight lag in movement and interprets the resulting signal to determine directional head movement and force.

Otoliths have a small amount of protein within their structure, and this protein's function is to help the otolith anchor adequately to the otolithic membrane. However, certain conditions can cause the otolith to become dislodged from the otolithic membrane. When this occurs, otoliths are allowed to move freely around the labyrinth system of the inner ear. The presence of these loose otoliths within the labyrinth is one of the main suspected causes of BPPV.

Detachment of otoliths from the otolithic membrane can occur in response to head trauma physically knocking the otoliths from the membrane. However, as only 15% of reported BPPV cases are due to head trauma, other mechanisms are capable of freeing the otoliths from the otolithic membrane. For example, it has been shown that otoliths degenerate over time, and this degeneration tends to increase with age[5]. This degeneration decreases the anchoring of the otolith to the otolithic membrane[6]. Consequently, otoliths in the process of degenerating can become dislodged from the otolithic membrane and be released into the endolymphatic space of the utricle or saccule in response to a very mild force[7]. Separately, it has been suggested that a change in the pH of the fluid within the labyrinth system may also contribute to allowing otoliths to detach from the otolithic membrane[8].

Semicircular Canals

In addition to the saccule and utricle, the three semicircular canals of the inner ear's labyrinth network make up the remainder of the vestibular system. And along with otoliths, these semicircular canals are suspected to have a high degree of involvement in BPPV.

Like the cochlea, the semicircular canals are formed by the surrounding bone which creates three 'tunnels' or canals through the temporal bone. Membranes snake through the bone-encased semicircular canals and serve to contain the endolymph within the labyrinth system. Like each maculi of the utricle and saccule, motions of the head cause the endolymph to move within the canals. As the movement of endolymph flows across specialized sensors, signals are sent to the brain which interpret the direction of head movement.

There are three independent semicircular canals that serve to provide feedback about head position. These three canals are designated the anterior, posterior, and horizontal canal. Based on their position, the three canals are effectively placed at right angles to each other which in turn allows all head motions to be detected. This design can be imagined by thinking of a corner of a cube – each of the three sides of the cube outlines a different plane of movement and are positioned at right angles to each other.

In terms of structure and function of the canals, the anterior canal is positioned higher than the other two canals and is responsible for detecting motions such as occur when nodding one's head. The horizontal canal is the shortest of the three canals and is responsible for detecting motion such as when turning the head to signal the motion of "no". The third canal is the posterior canal which sits lower than the other two canals and serves to detect motion such as might occur if you touch one of your ears to its same-side shoulder.

Whereas the saccule and utricle detect 'linear' movement such as acceleration or vertical movement, the semicircular canals detect 'angular' movement. An example of angular movement would be that occurring if turning the head side-to-side as if watching a tennis match. Because the movement does not generate forces that act upon the saccule or utricle, the design of the semicircular canals can detect this angular motion and provide feedback to the brain regarding the type of movement.

Detection of motion occurs as endolymph passes over specialized areas of each canal. Movement of the head causes movement of endolymph, which in turn flows across hair cells that moves in response to the pressure of the moving fluid. These hair cells are located within the canal itself, at each end of the semicircular canal in an area called the *ampulla* (see Figure 1.3). The ampulla is a bulged-out area of the semicircular canal near the utricle. Hair cells within the ampulla contain a gelatinous cover called the *cupula* that covers the hair cells and extends across the entire width of the semicircular canal.

As we discussed, when a person moves his or her head the endolymph moves within the semicircular canal in response to the head movement. As the fluid moves, it flows around the cupula (Figure 1.4). As the motion of the endolymph pushes against the cupula, the cupula bends. This causes hair cells immediately under the cupula to also bend, the same way a tree branch might bend if its leafy end were placed into flowing water. This bending of the hair cells sends a signal to the brain which is interpreted as motion appropriate to the direction of head movement.

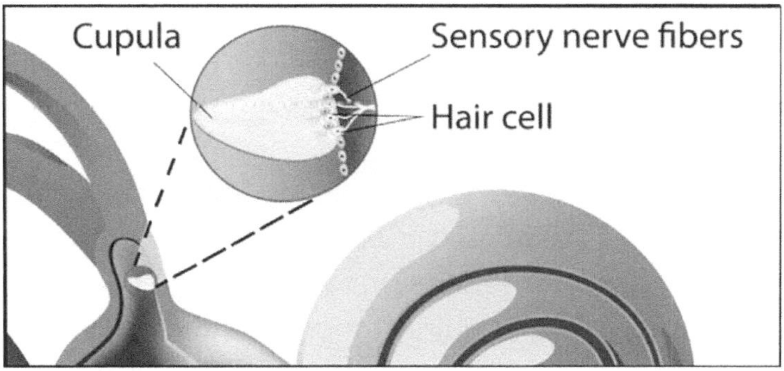

Figure 1.4. The cupula resides within the ampulla of each semicircular canal. Movement of endolymph causes the cupula to bend, thereby activating the underlying hair cells. Action of the cupula is suspected to be highly involved in BPPV.

These events occurring within the semicircular canals are important to understand, as they are involved in the two different types of BPPV. As far back as the 1960s, researchers believed that BPPV resulted from otoliths acting upon the cupula within the semicircular canal[9]. It was thought at the time that BPPV resulted from otoliths actually adhering to the cupula, in turn causing the cupula to become heavier and making it more sensitive to motion of the fluid within the semicircular canal[10]. As we will discuss in the next chapter, this effect of otoliths acting upon the cupula is still accepted even today.

Summary

Because BPPV involves a disruption to the structures of the inner ear, this chapter's introduction to the involved anatomy can help explain the underlying causes behind those symptoms involved in BPPV. Perhaps more importantly, outlining the anatomy of the labyrinth system can help explain why canalith repositioning procedures have proven to be highly effective at eliminating the symptoms of BPPV. Later, we will examine these repositioning procedures and highlight how the maneuvers are used to move the otoliths out of the semicircular canals and back into the utricle. But first we will discuss what BPPV is specific to its history, the involved anatomy, relevant terminology, and how it affects the population.

Chapter 2: What is BPPV?

DESPITE ITS IMPOSING name, BPPV is a relatively common condition of the inner ear that invokes a sensation of spinning in response to certain head positions[11]. Each word in the name of the condition serves to outline a specific component of BPPV. *Benign* represents the non-harmful effects of BPPV, indicating that it is not a serious or life-threatening condition. *Paroxysmal* characterizes the sudden and forceful nature of the symptoms of BPPV such as vertigo and nystagmus. *Positional* outlines that BPPV occurs when the head is placed in certain positions. And perhaps the most well-known term, *vertigo,* details the sensation of spinning which may induce a loss of balance. Placed together, the words used in naming BPPV represent that it is a relatively harmless condition that brings on rapid and strong vertigo in response to certain positions of the head.

Benign paroxysmal positional vertigo has been called by many different names. "Benign positional vertigo", "paroxysmal positional vertigo", "positional vertigo", "benign paroxysmal nystagmus", or "paroxysmal positional nystagmus" have all been used, but the most commonly used term remains *benign positional paroxysmal vertigo*[12]. Vertigo has been defined as the sensation of self-motion (of head/body) when no self-motion is occurring, or the sensation of distorted self-motion during an otherwise normal head movement[13]. The word 'positional' has come under more scrutiny, however. Some researchers have suggested that the word *positional* be replaced with *positioning*, as BPPV occurs in response to the head being moved to a new position[14]. These researchers argue that *positional* indicates that the effects of BPPV are based on holding the head in a certain position, when in fact the act of moving the head (i.e. *positioning)* is what actually triggers the effects. Nevertheless, the Bárány Society in 2015 released the "Consensus document of the Committee for the Classification of Vestibular Disorders" which solidified use of the term *positional*[14].

BPPV has been called the most common vestibular disorder[15]. One study of 590 patients evaluated for dizziness found BPPV to be the underlying cause of the dizziness 33.9% of the time, more than ten percent higher than the next leading cause[16]. Often, the first event of vertigo associated with BPPV is reported to occur in bed or when getting out of bed[17]. And, the vertigo occurs each time the patient's head is placed in a specific position, which may occur in conjunction with performing a particular movement such as looking upwards[17]. If the head position is maintained, the vertigo usually continues for a while before gradually coming to a stop (i.e. 'fatiguing vertigo'). Conversely, if the vertigo begins but then the head position is immediately changed, the vertigo typically stops.

When the vertigo is not occurring as a result of certain head positions, most patients report no lingering symptoms and as such, patients typically report no issues with normal daily activities such as walking, driving a car, or exercising. Other patients, however, report dizziness when walking during periods of BPPV-associated flare-ups[18]. Still others report a feeling of floating, and express some degree of unsteadiness even when the attacks are not occurring[17].

A brief history of BPPV

As far back as the 1920s, BPPV was thought to involve small crystals of the inner ear. Robert Barany described the first patient with BPPV in 1921[17] and outlined that symptoms were likely due to abnormal otoliths[11]. In the 1950s, a procedure termed the Dix-Hallpike test was able to specifically elicit the conditions of BPPV, lending further evidence to a cause. Margaret Dix and Charles Hallpike found that the nystagmus 'fatigued' in many patients when their test was repeated. Furthermore, a response lagged about five seconds behind any positioning, with elimination of the symptoms if the patient sits upright[19]. Their findings eventually led them to determine that BPPV is a condition of the labyrinth, specifically the utricular macula[19].

In the 1960s, physical evidence was found that began to explain the reason for the positional vertigo. Schuknecht found material within the semicircular canals of the ear in BPPV patients and suggested that this material therefore became more sensitive to gravity, in turn triggering the effects that BPPV patients experience. However, it was noted that Schuknecht's theory didn't explain the transient nature of BPPV, as many patients outlined that their vertigo resolved itself relatively soon despite no change in head position.

By the early 1980s, Hall had outlined a new mechanism for BPPV which again outlined particles within the ear as the source of BPPV[20]. Evidence for this particle theory stemmed from finding clusters of calcium-carbonate crystals (i.e. otoliths) within the semicircular canals during surgery performed on patients affected by BPPV[21].

This theory was later solidified by Epley, who in 1992 released a study detailing the outcomes of his repositioning procedure which relieved BPPV in 90-97% of patients[20]. Interestingly, despite overwhelming success in using his maneuvers to eliminate the symptoms of BPPV, Dr. Epley's techniques were initially met with strong resistance from the medical community, due in part to a rather simple fix for what had previously been assumed to be a very complex problem. Over time, however, Dr. Epley's efforts became more accepted, and the repositioning procedure eventually became named after Dr. Epley. Since its development in the early 1990's, the Epley maneuver has undergone a few further modifications to get it to the point at which it exists today.

Epidemiology of BPPV

Epidemiology is the study of how a disease or condition affects the health of various populations. Looking at the epidemiology of BPPV can help us understand how common the condition is, who it affects, and potentially how it affects certain individuals. What the research has shown us is that of all disorders related to equilibrium, BPPV accounts for approximately 15%[22]. While this may seem like a relatively low amount (i.e. less than one in five equilibrium disorders are from BPPV), it should be noted that in adults, BPPV is the most common cause of vertigo[17], affecting between 17-42% of patients evaluated for vertigo[23]. In other words, BPPV, despite its sometimes overwhelming effects, is a relatively common condition.

Specific to gender, women experience BPPV approximately twice as much as men[17]. However, no known reason for the higher occurrence in women has been reported. There does appear to be a genetic predisposition for BPPV, as patients with BPPV are five times more likely to have a relative with BPPV[24]. In other words, if a sibling or parent has BPPV, it is much more likely that another individual in the family will experience BPPV as well. Furthermore, being affected by other ear conditions can also increase one's risk for having BPPV, as research indicates that BPPV is more common in patients who have had vestibular neuritis[17] as well as Ménière's[25].

While it is possible that there is a yet-undiscovered genetic component that makes certain individuals more susceptible to be afflicted with BPPV, approximately 15% of BPPV cases result from some sort of trauma in the area of the head. As discussed in Chapter 1, the temporal bone – which houses the semicircular canals – is very dense and can directly transfer traumatic forces to the otolith organs. However traumatic force is not required, as both whiplash and high-impact exercise have been shown to trigger BPPV[17], along with reports of BPPV occurring after surgery[17].

The lifetime prevalence – or percent of the population that has had BPPV at some point in their life – has been reported to be 2.4%[26]. Similarly, the lifetime risk, or chance that *any* individual will experience BPPV at some point in their life, is 10%[27]. These values are relatively high for a medical condition and reflect how BPPV is somewhat common in the population. As an individual ages, the chance of experiencing BPPV increases, with the peak age range for developing BPPV being between 50 and 60 years of age[28]. This age range also reflects the fact that BPPV is very rare in children[27].

Interestingly, evidence suggests that BPPV is more common than reported. The prevalence of undiagnosed BPPV is relatively high. Evidence for this stems in part from one study that looked at nearly 200 young adults who were not being treated for dizziness. They found a prevalence of BBPV within this group of 9% using positional assessment[29]. Ironically, this 9% prevalence was the same exact rate a separate study found in a group of 100 geriatric patients[30]. These findings suggest that almost one in 10 people have undiagnosed BPPV.

Recurrence of BPPV

Though BPPV is often treated with a single visit to a trained medical professional, it can reoccur. In fact, approximately half of patients with BPPV suffer an eventual recurrence of BPPV within three years[31], with most of the reoccurrences happening within the first year. In other words, up to half of people that experience BPPV and then recover fully will have a second episode in the future. Interestingly, the recurrence rate for BPPV is higher when BPPV results from trauma than from idiopathic (i.e. 'spontaneous') causes[32, 33]. When the recurrent attacks continue over time, the frequency of the attacks vary from patient to patient, with some patients having attacks spaced closely together while others report being symptom-free for years before another vertigo attack hits[17]. Logically, one might expect that the recurrent episode occurs in the same ear; however, about one fourth of recurrences of BPPV occur in the *opposite* ear[34]. This suggests that there may be some sort of anatomical anomaly that predisposes the otoliths to become dislodged in a particular individual.

One possible explanation for the relatively high (~50%) rate of recurrence focuses on an involvement of calcium in otolith development. For example, one study found an association between BPPV and its rate of recurrence among individuals with calcium metabolism dysfunction and vitamin D deficiency[35, 36]. This suggests that decreased levels of calcium and/or vitamin D may play a role in making otoliths more susceptible to detachment, in turn allowing the otoliths to work their way more easily into the semicircular canals in some individuals.

It is important to note that one or two recurrent episodes of BPPV that arise after successful repositioning procedures (e.g. Epley maneuver) should not be considered abnormal. However, persistent BPPV that does not respond to repositioning can be problematic, and as we will discuss later actually falls under a more serious condition known as "intractable BPPV". Intractable BPPV is not typically a minor condition like BPPV can be. Rather, it often causes significant issues for the patient as the vertigo is not easily fixed like typically occurs with traditional BPPV. We will discuss the differences between BPPV and intractable BPPV in the next chapter.

Alongside cases involving recurrence of BPPV, spontaneous remission of BPPV can also occur in some individuals. Spontaneous remission of BPPV occurs when the symptoms associated with BPPV resolve without any therapeutic intervention, and has been reported to take anywhere from 17-39 days for the posterior canal BPPV and 7-16 days for BPPV originating in the horizontal-canal[28, 37]. Others have reported that spontaneous relief of BPPV occurs within one month in 20% of patients, and within three months in 50% of patients[38].

Location of BPPV in the inner ear

Of the three canals in the ear, BPPV is most commonly found in one of two canals. The posterior semicircular canal is most often affected, occurring in up to 95% of cases[22, 39]. However, a bit of variation exists in various literature reports, including studies indicating that approximately 15-20% of BPPV cases involve the lateral canal[12, 17, 27]. The higher frequency of BPPV within the posterior semicircular canal is thought to be due to its gravity-dependent positioning[22], meaning that the posterior canal's design, coupled with the force of gravity, makes it a natural location for free otoliths to gather. Interestingly, the right ear's posterior canal is the most commonly-involved side, thought to result from people sleeping more often on their right side[40].

Because BPPV is not limited to occurrence within one particular semicircular canal, movements that initiate symptoms can vary between patients. For example, my own BPPV-associated vertigo occurred when looking straight up with my head was slightly tilted to the right. Vertigo in association with this head position was a clear indication of posterior canal involvement, based upon those movements that triggered my vertigo. If I brought my head back to a normal position, the vertigo stopped immediately. Similarly, someone who reports vertigo occurring when rolling sideways, such as might occur during a 'logroll' or when turning over in bed, could be expected to have BPPV associated with the lateral canal.

Symptoms of BPPV

For most patients affected by BPPV, they report brief attacks of vertigo combined with nystagmus that occurs in response to changes in head position[37]. The most commonly reported symptom of BPPV is dizziness that is triggered by head movement[7]. A short, forceful sensation of vertigo occurs next, along with likely feelings of imbalance even when head movements are avoided[7]. Other symptoms exist with BPPV but are less consistent between patients. These symptoms include rotational vertigo (in 86% of patients), oscillopsia (31%), nausea (33%), vomiting (14%), imbalance (49%), fear of falling (36%), and falls (1%)[27].

Whereas the primary symptom of vertigo occurs rapidly during a bout of BPPV, along with possible nausea and vomiting in some cases, the initial experience of BPPV can be quite psychologically traumatic for a patient. Thoughts of epilepsy, stroke, or other serious head conditions are not uncommon, and it is certainly understandable given the forceful series of events that BPPV can bring.

The source behind the symptoms of BPPV are somewhat unique from those of many other medical conditions in that they are suspected to occur in response to physical disruption of one of the body's sensors. Often times, symptoms such as pain result when a part of the body is damaged or loses its function, such as may occur in response to a traumatic injury. As we have outlined previously, BPPV results not necessarily from damage to a particular part of the body but rather because specific nerves are being activated inadvertently by small, displaced calcium crystals making their way into a highly sensitive portion of one of the semicircular canals. Despite the sometimes forceful symptoms associated with BPPV, simply moving those crystals back to their intended location typically results in immediate cessation of symptoms. It's unlikely that any other medical condition has as strong of symptoms that can be so quickly and easily eliminated as those associated with BPPV.

Cause of BPPV

It is now well-accepted that BPPV results from otolith material becoming detached and making its way into one or more of the semicircular canals[17]. Evidence for this comes from direct observation of otolith material within the semicircular canals of patients with BPPV[21]. Once the otoliths have made their way into the semicircular canals, they are free to move around the endolymph. Interestingly, research has shown that detached otoliths should dissolve in the endolymph, but evidence suggests that the calcium concentration of the endolymph can prevent otoliths from dissolving in some individuals[41].

It is important to note that it's not necessarily *any* amount of free-floating otoliths being in the semicircular canals that cause BPPV, as a small amount of otoliths being present within the canals at any time is rather common. Instead, it is hypothesized that a significant build-up of otoliths is necessary to produce enough force to bend the cupula[42]. Therefore, having otoliths within one's semicircular canal does not necessarily mean that the individual will have BPPV. In fact, one study found that of ten people who had otoliths present within their semicircular canals, only one reported BPPV prior to examination[42].

Once in a semicircular canal, the otoliths are at the mercy of gravity and tend to always settle at the lowest point found in association with a particular head position. Because of the design of the semicircular canals, head movement in certain directions can move the otoliths within the endolymph to a point where they contact the sensory nerves of the vestibular system. By activating these nerves to a greater degree than what normally occurs, it is thought to provide a sensation of movement even though the head remains still[17]. This is the sensation we experience as 'vertigo'.

There are two current types of BPPV, and both are initiated within the semicircular canal. As we discussed in the previous chapter, the cupula extends into the semicircular canal and detects the movement of endolymph flowing around the cupula. The cupula itself is sensitive to fluid pressure that occurs when the endolymph effectively presses against it. However, when the heavier otoliths move through the semicircular canal and contact the cupula, the nerves of the cupula are stimulated to a greater degree, thereby causing the brain to receive 'excess signaling' which is interpreted as excess head movement. When the otoliths are thought to be adhering to the cupula and triggering vertigo and nystagmus, the type of BPPV is referred to as *cupulolithiasis* (e.g. "heavy cupula").

The cupulolithiasis theory of BPPV was thought to be the sole cause of BPPV for over 30 years. Eventually, however, it was realized that cupulolithiasis could not explain how in some types of BPPV, the vertigo dissipated on its own after a short time (i.e. "fatiguing" vertigo) even if the head position was maintained. If otoliths did indeed attach or adhere to the cupula to make it heavier, the cupula should be expected to remain activated in certain head positions, in turn causing continuous vertigo rather than fatiguing vertigo[11]. Therefore, a second theory outlining a cause for BPPV eventually developed.

This second suspected cause of BPPV was termed canalolithiasis (i.e. "moving otoconia"). In this theory, free (unattached) otoliths build up within the semicircular canals. Because the semicircular canals are designed to be sensitive to the movement of fluid, the additional mass of the otoliths causes irregular motion of the endolymph in the semicircular canal. This in turn causes the cupula to be abnormally stimulated[14]. The movement of unattached otoliths within the semicircular canals, combined with particular head positions that move the otoliths up against the cupula, is thought to be the reason why vertigo is typically transient (i.e. fades over time) in BPPV.

The type of BPPV a person is experiencing (canalolithiasis vs cupulolithiasis) can be determined by evaluating the symptoms that are reported by the patient, specifically the type of nystagmus that is elicited. Canalolithiasis-based nystagmus is the most common type, lasting less than one minute in total duration and often exhibiting latency (i.e. taking a few seconds to occur) after the triggering head position is reached[10]. Cupulolithiasis, on the other hand, is relatively instant in its occurrence and can last longer than a minute.

Summary

As we have outlined in this chapter, BPPV is a relatively common yet highly intricate medical condition. Although the specific type of BPPV can vary, the symptoms are generally the same in that certain positions of the head can trigger vertigo and nystagmus, along with other potential conditions.

For the vast majority of patients, relief from BPPV can occur with a single office visit that utilizes one of several different repositioning maneuvers to move the offending otoliths back into a different area of the inner ear. Unfortunately, not all patients are fully cured of BPPV after repositioning maneuvers. Many of these individuals must undergo much more invasive procedures due to a condition called "intractable BPPV". In the next chapter, we'll look at this condition as well as the available treatments that can help fix BPPV that does not respond to traditional treatment techniques.

Chapter 3: Intractable BPPV

FOR THE OVERWHELMING majority of patients, BPPV can be fixed using one of several available repositioning maneuvers. Thanks to these repositioning procedures, symptoms associated with BPPV that may have been present for years can literally be eliminated in just a minute or two, often with no lingering reminders that it ever existed. It is not uncommon for some patients to have a recurrence of BPPV over the years, but for most individuals, once the repositioning procedures remove the otoliths from the semicircular canals, the effects of BPPV are gone for good.

Other individuals, however, either do not respond to repositioning maneuvers – even when the maneuvers are repeated several times – or have frequent, recurring episodes of BPPV that continue to 'flare up' despite seemingly successful repositioning. These individuals are said to be suffering from a more severe form of BPPV known as *intractable* (i.e. "hard to deal with", or "stubborn") BPPV.

Whereas simple non-invasive attempts such as Epley's maneuvers have no effect on an intractable BPPV patient's vertigo, invasive intervention techniques including the injection of medicine as well as surgery may be necessary to alleviate symptoms.

Epidemiology of Intractable BPPV

Patients with intractable BPPV are considered those who have either "persistent BPPV" that continues even with physical therapy of up to one year[10, 43], or "recurrent BPPV" that consists of frequent relapses after previous symptoms had disappeared[10]. Research indicates that persistent BPPV can occur in up to 12.5% of patients, and recurrent BPPV occurs at up to 10-25% of BPPV patients[44]. Risk factors for the development of intractable BPPV include an individual being age 50 or above, head trauma, and additional conditions including diabetes, hypertension, osteoporosis, or vitamin D deficiency, among others[10].

Causes of Intractable BPPV

Research from the 1990s reported that intractable BPPV is most likely due to one of three likely causes[45]. These three causes included improperly performed canalith repositioning, cupulolithiasis, and an obstruction within the posterior canal itself. More recently, several causes of intractable BPPV have been reported. These causes include osteoporosis, trauma, sleeping position, diabetes, and Ménière's disease[46].

An additional explanation for intractable BPPV involving apogeotropic nystagmus (i.e. rapid eye movement toward the ceiling) has been termed *undetachable cupulolithiasis*, in which the otoliths have essentially adhered to the cupula and thereby do not respond to treatment[47]. Others have shown that patients with intractable BPPV are more likely to have abnormal canals than patients without intractable BPPV[46]. Conditions associated with the abnormal canal included a narrowing of the canal (i.e. stenosis) as well as a blockage resulting from otolith debris. The researchers suggested that the narrowing of the canal could be the cause of any blockage which in turn becomes non-responsive to normal positioning treatment.

While intractable BPPV can cause severe disruption of daily life, the condition itself may actually occur less frequently than previously thought. Research has found that many people who were previously diagnosed as having intractable BPPV were simply misdiagnosed as having posterior canal BPPV when they really had BPPV within a different canal[43]. Therefore, these patients stood no chance of benefitting from treatment, as that treatment was focused on BPPV originating from the posterior canal BPPV.

Treatment of Intractable BPPV

Intratympanic Methylprednisolone

Medication is generally not used for the treatment of traditional BPPV given the consistently favorable results associated with repositioning procedures as well as the positional nature of BPPV. However, intractable BPPV occurs when the positioning procedures have failed and other more invasive methods must be utilized. Recently, one study reported the benefit of injecting the anti-inflammatory medication methylprednisolone directly into the middle ear. Researchers found that seven out of nine individuals who failed to get relief after at least six repositioning attempts did report improvement after injection of methylprednisolone.

Furthermore, none of those reporting benefits from the injection had any further incidents of vertigo during follow-up[48].

Betahistine is a drug used for the treatment of nausea and motion sickness which causes an increase of blood flow within the inner ear. One study found that among patients with BPPV, combining canalith repositioning (i.e. Epley's maneuver) with betahistine resulted in less relapse of BPPV symptoms[49]. Although patients in this study were not noted to have intractable BPPV, the fact that recurrence of BPPV was diminished in these patients suggests that those with intractable BPPV may also have a reduction in recurrence rate, though the actual recurrence rate needs to be tested specifically in this population.

Neurectomy

Surgical intervention for intractable BPPV typically involves one of two procedures. The first procedure involves nerve transection (i.e. 'cutting') of the posterior ampullary nerve of the ear, sometimes referred to as the "singular" nerve. Normally, this nerve is responsible for sending signals from the posterior canal to the central nervous system in order to indicate movement of the head. Research indicates that 96% of patients with intractable BPPV were cured of vertigo after surgical cutting of this nerve, and only 7% suffered some degree of hearing loss[50].

It is typical for patients to exhibit vertigo upon the actual cutting of the nerve and report dizziness for a few days after the surgical procedure. As noted above, some degree of patients report no relief in symptoms after nerve transection, but this lack of relief has been attributed to factors such as an incorrect diagnosis (i.e. the wrong semicircular canal) or incomplete cutting of the nerve[43].

Semicircular Canal occlusion

The second surgical procedure used for intractable BPPV is known as posterior canal occlusion. For this procedure, the posterior canal is filled using a 'plug' of bone recovered from the surgical process and held in place using a special glue[51]. Preventing the flow of endolymph within an affected canal has the effect of inhibiting movement of the ampulla within the offending semicircular canal. Consequently, inability of the ampulla to send signals from a malfunctioning canal results in no abnormal signals being sent to the brain which would normally trigger vertigo for the patient. Because only one of the two posterior canals are typically affected, the healthy canal that contains no otoliths takes over after the occlusive procedure and the patient eventually returns to a normal lifestyle.

The success of posterior canal occlusion at relieving the vertigo associated with intractable BPPV can exceed 90%[52] and has even been reported to be 100% successful[50]. Furthermore, hearing is typically maintained with this procedure[53]. However, some patients who have undergone posterior canal occlusion have reported short-term hearing loss as well as dizziness for up to six weeks after the procedure. In rare cases, permanent hearing loss has been reported[52]. Research from one particular study found that 94 of 97 patients on whom this procedure was performed experienced complete relief of vertigo after a relatively short period (two days to a few weeks) of dizziness. Four individuals experienced hearing loss, but this included hearing loss due to post-surgical infection as well as unintentional drilling on the incus bone of the middle ear[43].

Summary

Intractable BPPV is much more serious and more involved than traditional BPPV. Because intractable BPPV does not respond to treatment, patients are often left at the mercy of the condition, subjecting them to extended periods of vertigo, nystagmus, and possibly nausea in response to certain head positions. Particularly frustrating for these individuals is that the cause – free otoliths – is generally the same as traditional BPPV, yet the repositioning maneuvers used to treat BPPV are relatively ineffective in the long term for intractable BPPV. As such, more invasive, permanent interventions are often needed when treating intractable BPPV, though they can be quite successful at reducing the symptoms of BPPV.

Chapter 4: My story

MY OWN INTERACTION with BPPV was also my first experience in what I would term a 'non-traditional' medical condition. I've had broken bones, pulled muscles, sore joints, and the like, but those were easily recognizable medical conditions with not only a clear onset but also a predictable healing timeframe. So, once inflicted with the effects of BPPV my mindset was forced to change. I had no idea what was occurring, and the effects of the condition were not like anything I had ever felt before. This unfamiliarity led to paranoid thoughts and quite a bit of stress, though I later learned that the effects of BPPV were in fact quite minimal. But how I learned the relatively harmless nature of BPPV required quite a long journey in itself.

In 2001 at the age of 26 I began practicing a sport called Brazilian Jiu Jitsu (BJJ). I had fallen in love with the art a few years earlier while watching videos of the new sport of mixed martial arts, but had not been able to take up the sport earlier due to a lack of either finances or a locale. Finally, while living in southeast Texas I had posted one day on a message board that I was looking to train in ground fighting in order to learn self-defense. Someone saw my post and recommended that I come with him to observe a BJJ class. By the end of the first class, I was hooked. The fascination I found in BJJ soon led me down a road that allowed me to not only improve my fitness but also improve my confidence in my ability to protect myself in the event is was needed.

A year in I was doing well. I took second place in my first-ever tournament and was extremely proud the day I received my blue belt, the second of five belts in the BJJ belt ranking system. I was doing great, and trying to get as much training in as my job would allow. One night, I took up an offer for an 'open call' for training, meaning that it wasn't an official class but rather an impromptu session. If anyone showed up, they would get to train. Upon arriving I found that it was only myself and the classmate who put out the call. Since he was higher-trained than me, it quickly turned in to an instructional lesson for me as he began showing me some techniques that had worked for him.

At one point I was lying on my back during a break. When the break was over, we decided to continue with the previous technique that we had been working on. This involved him being positioned at my side near my shoulders and applying a 'choke'. As he fell to his knees to get into position, he evidently misjudged his distance as his knee slammed against the side of my head. It was painful, but as I was lying down on my back there was really no better position for me, so I remained on my back to try and let the pain dissipate.

Suddenly, I felt a tremendous sensation inside my head. It was like my brain had been dropped against the side of my skull or something, with a twinge of feeling somewhat like my brain was being electrocuted. It was an overpowering sensation and one that I could not ignore. Strange? Yes. Frightening? Absolutely. I shot up from the floor all the way to my feet. I started pacing rapidly. My classmate was still on his knees, wondering what was happening. I remember shaking my head, saying 'no' non-verbally but more intending to imply 'leave me alone for a minute'.

Strangely, the issue was gone as soon as it had appeared. When walking around I was almost normal, save for the lingering symptoms resulting from the trauma of his knee hitting against my head. I brushed it off almost as if it hadn't happened.

"Perhaps it was some complication of the knee to my head" I told myself. I'd never had severe head trauma before, so I rationalized that I just didn't know what a minor concussion felt like. But because it was gone so quickly, and because I felt relatively normal, I felt I could go on. So I laid back down to continue the technique.

WHAM! It hit again. And I shot up to my feet again. It was an incredible feeling. Not painful, just extremely frightening and somewhat violent at the same time. This time, I walked outside and down the stairs. My training partner was left clueless, not understanding the symptoms nor the complete confusion I was feeling at the moment. He stepped outside to ask me if I was OK, but all I could do was utter a mumbling "I don't know" or some similar non-specific response. My intended message was that something wasn't right and I needed to be left alone. After all, how exactly do you describe something that doesn't hurt and disappears quickly? I wasn't sure what to think now, because once again the sensations were gone as soon as I stood up.

Needless to say, the training ended there for the night. I was a nervous wreck, and my training partner didn't need the constant interruptions. I drove the 25 miles home wondering both what the heck happened as well as *did that just happen*? Since there were no lingering symptoms I had no record of anything actually having occurred. So, I began to question myself as to what occurred, and whether I had misinterpreted some muscle strain or other minor injury. In the end, I blew it off and decided that I'd just resume training at the next scheduled class. In my mind, the incident never happened.

The next morning I went to take a shower as I had done every morning for pretty much my entire adult life. I turned my back to the shower head and slowly began turning my head back and forth to get my hair wet. That's when it happened. BANG! The sensation returned with a vengeance, and I collapsed in the shower, nearly taking down the shower curtain with me. Confused, a bit annoyed, and somewhat scared, I slowly looked up and noticed again that the sensation had stopped. Not knowing what was happening, I repeated the motion of my head in the shower. BANG! Again.

Now I was beginning to get some data about what was happening. When my head was tilted back and to the side – just like the previous night while lying on the floor, the sensation hit. I tried other head positions but to no avail. However, if I laid on my bed, looked up, and turned my head to the right – I was instantly informed that I had found the 'magic' position. As I repeatedly caused the sensation to occur, I began isolating what was happening. My vision started to shake, followed by a strange shaking sensation within my head as well. The shaky vision effect slowly worsened until I could see nothing as a result of the rapid motion of my eyes causing everything to be a blur.

I eventually stood up and replicated the motion of my head as when I had been in the shower. Once again, I had a successful elicitation of the vertigo effect. What I noticed was that if I tipped my head back and to the right, such that my left ear was almost pointing up, I could elicit the response. Strangely, the *bang* effect that happened initially had disappeared and I was left only with a slow (three to four second) onset which eventually turned into a phase of rapid eye movements that completely blurred my vision. I found that if I held the position long enough, the effects would slowly fade after 30 seconds or so. I kept repeating the movement, trying to understand what was going on inside my head. I had medical training, but my specialty was in orthopedics – joints and muscles. I knew that this wasn't a neck problem, and I was clueless as to why my eyes were acting the way that they were.

Around that time, the internet had begun to grow immensely. We were past the dot-com bubble bursting, but medical information hadn't quite grown to the level we know it today. So, my attempts to find a reason for the strange sensations went unanswered in my searches. After a few days, I accepted the reality of what was going on, and assumed that it would pass similar to any other strange malady I'd had previously. Over the next few weeks, which turned into months, the sensations remained with little sign of dissipating. I kept testing the 'status' of the sensations by spending much of my day tilting my head back, having no clue as to what was causing this incredibly powerful series of events.

Eventually, I accepted that this strange new condition was going to stick around for a while. I learned which head and body positions triggered the symptoms and became adept at avoiding those positions. For example, laying on my back in bed was fine, but if I looked over at my alarm clock I would have to do it quickly before the sensations set in. Other times, I would purposely cause the strange events just to see if they were getting worse, staying the same, or improving. Unfortunately, I had no change in symptoms over time. Five months in, I was starting to accept that I was stuck with this. Perhaps it was one of those "growing old" things I had heard about, even though I was only 27 at the time. Regardless, I adapted. I had been back at BJJ and performing relatively well with no real issues. I showered differently now. And I was more cognizant of my body position when in bed.

One day I happened to be at my physician's office having a casual conversation when I mentioned to him what I had been feeling. My physician was also a friend of mine, so I saw him on a social basis much more than I saw him for medical reasons. I told him I had been having some dizziness and that it only appeared when I put my head in a certain position. I tilted my head back and felt the strange sensations. Popping my head back up, I saw the odd look in his eyes as if to say *you're weird.* However, I then asked him to come stand by me, which he did. I asked him to watch my eyes, and then tilted my head back. As the crazy eye movement started, he let out a "whoa", to which I quickly returned my head to upright and smugly confirmed my earlier comment. He thought about it for a moment, then went over to his books. Reading through a couple of conditions, he came across one called *benign positional paroxysmal vertigo.*

Reading the symptoms off, I knew quickly that he had found my condition. All I wanted at that point was to make it stop, and asked him how to go about doing just that. He kept reading, describing a repositioning procedure, to which I was oblivious but eager to take on.

My next stop was to a local audiologist. There, I described my symptoms and was eager to get the process underway. I underwent a barrage of tests that included following a series of red dots on the wall and an annoying mix of hot and cold water being injected in my ear. Then, I was subjected to a series of positional moves while wearing what I will describe as 'unique' glasses, which actually held a camera that would record my eye movement during the positional changes.

You know that you have got something exclusive going on when a medical professional elicits a "whoa" during your testing. The audiologist mentioned that she had never observed as forceful of eye movement during the positional head changes as my eyes revealed. I knew that my eyes went crazy when I elicited the symptoms myself, but to hear that it was the worst a professional had ever encountered seemed strangely gratifying. In a way, her revealing that told me that this wasn't all in my head, and that I had a legitimate reason for feeling like something wasn't right.

The head positioning tests provided her the information she needed. She explained to me, as my physician first proposed, that I had a condition called BPPV, or benign positional paroxysmal vertigo. My questioning look brought about by such a strange name was quickly erased when she informed me of what was going on, and that it was relatively common. I learned that I had small crystals in my ear that had been knocked loose and were floating around my ear until they reached a nerve, at which point they would trigger some sort of response in the nerve which for me resulted in the rapid eye movement. I asked her what we needed to do to get rid of it, and she said it is successfully treated with a very similar procedure of head positioning as I had just experienced during the testing. I was all in.

The day of the 'repositioning', I was instructed to bring someone with me as I would not be able to drive home. I was at this point skeptical of the procedures, as it seemed a little too easy to stop such a violent response with a little 'rolling around' on a table. But, I was willing to try.

As the procedure started, she started a timer in order to hold my head in each position for a specific amount of time. As we began, the timer abruptly fell onto the floor. With my head in her hands and a protocol to follow, she quickly started yelling for an assistant to get the timer, all the while afraid to stop the procedure for fear of negating the effects of the treatment. Eventually, calm was restored as the timer was recovered, allowing the procedure to continue.

As I sat up upon completion of the repositioning, I was fitted with a soft cervical collar and instructed to maintain an upright position for 48 hours. *What about sleep*, I thought. She soon informed me that sleeping would need to be done in the upright position, a posture that I am not successful in getting much sleep in. Despite her instructions, all I wanted to do was tilt my head back and see if I was free of the annoying *nystagmus*, as she had termed my rapid eye movement. Doing this however, was forbidden as she explained that it would increase the risk of the crystals moving back into the canals of my inner ear. I was stuck – maintaining a vertical posture for the next 48 hours or risking a return visit for another 48 hour attempt.

Upon arriving home I figured that I would make the most of my vertical posture and surf the internet for what info I could about BPPV. The results were highly favorable, indicating that most individuals who go through the positioning that I did were asymptomatic within days. I felt relieved, yet somewhat perturbed that I would have to maintain this position for two more days. Still, I wanted to tilt my head back . . . just to check. But I abstained.

That night I struggled to get comfortable in bed. It's hard to position yourself so that your head is vertical without requiring that your lower spine is also vertical. You don't realize how easy it is to tilt your head back until you're told that you are not allowed to do so. So I had to position my pillows in a way that my back was flat yet my upper spine curved enough to allow my neck and head to remain vertical. In other words, I created the world's worst posture setup.

Sleep was difficult, but it happened eventually. When I awoke, however, I was shocked to find that I had reversed my body 180 degrees. My head was still vertical, but somehow my chest was against the pillows. It was strange indeed, but yet I was relieved that I appeared to have survived any non-vertical positioning. The rest of the day was relatively uneventful, as it is not hard to remain upright with an excessively large, overly soft neck brace wrapped around your throat. I remember counting down the hours – both the hours until I had to go back to sleep, and the hours until this neck brace ordeal was over. This whole crazy process just had to work, as I would not survive at work while wearing this neck brace and at the same time couldn't afford to take off an additional two days to repeat the procedure.

Eventually, nightfall came and I headed back to bed. I had created quite a framework of pillows on my bed, but I found out later that it worked, as I somehow woke up in the same position as I had fallen asleep in. Six more hours of the excessively vertical posture went off without a hitch. At 1pm, I unstrapped the neck brace and mentally prepared myself for the next step. I slowly tilted my head back and to the right and started my three-second countdown as I awaited the symptoms. Three . . . two . . . one . . . hmm . . . negative one? Negative two? Nothing. No nystagmus, no rattling in my brain. My BPPV was gone.

A part of me wanted to flop around on the bed. Another part of me wanted to go stand backwards in the shower and wet my hair in a way that I had not been allowed to do for the past several months. My better judgement kicked in and reminded me to not push my luck. At best, I was cured. At worst, the nystagmus and vertigo would return and I'd be subjected to two more days of living as if I were a telephone pole. I had no reason to risk it. So, I went about my day, only pausing every ten minutes or so to give a quick head tilt to check as well as to confirm. And I confirmed it, time after time. My BPPV was gone.

Chapter 5: Testing and Treatment of BPPV

SEVERAL CONDITIONS OF the ear can cause symptoms such as dizziness and vertigo that are typically associated with BPPV. These conditions range in severity and duration, and can include anything from a minor ear infection to much more serious conditions such as vestibular neuritis or Ménière's disease. Because many conditions can replicate the symptoms of BPPV it is essential that you are evaluated by a specialist trained in recognizing the numerous conditions of the inner ear. Though BPPV is relatively harmless in the long term, other conditions can worsen over time, and prompt treatment can help lessen the potential effects.

This chapter outlines the tests used to diagnose and treat BPPV. Because BPPV is thought to involve otoliths of the ear becoming displaced into the semicircular canals, diagnostic testing involves moving the head in a specific way that elicits the symptoms. Similarly, treatment of BPPV also involves specific positioning of the head, but includes moving the head through a series of precise positions that will cause the otoliths to travel from the affected semicircular canal back to the utricle area. Although the positional tests discussed in this chapter are well-established and widely available, it is important that patients experiencing dizziness discuss their symptoms with their physician so as to isolate a cause.

Diagnosis of BPPV

Despite its relatively common occurrence, BPPV is not easily recognized in a primary care setting[54]. Therefore, it is important that an affected individual be evaluated by a medical professional trained in recognizing inner ear disorders. Incorrect diagnoses can lead to prolonged delays in treatment, thereby sustaining a patient's reduced quality of life. Given the unique combination of sometimes severe symptoms as well as a relatively simple and inexpensive fix, proper diagnosis of BPPV is essential.

Due to the success of the many positioning methods involved in diagnostic testing for BPPV, the use of imaging (e.g. MRI, x-ray, etc.) is not typically required for patients exhibiting classic symptoms of

BPPV[12]. Specialized equipment could be used, such as a vibrating tool to help provide a physical force to move the otoliths within the semicircular canal, but this is most often not necessary.

The use of visual-recording glasses can often help provide a clear observation of the patient's nystagmus that occurs during the testing procedure[14]. Whereas movement of the head occurs along the same plane of movement as a particular semicircular canal being tested[17], recording the motion of the eyes in conjunction with a specific head movement can identify which semicircular canal is affected. Furthermore, the direction, intensity, duration, and latency of the nystagmus during testing provide important clues as to the location of the affected canal.

Given that there are three individual semicircular canals of the ear, it is possible that otoliths can be dislodged into any of the canals. As we have discussed, up to 95% of BPPV cases involve the posterior canal, with the remaining cases generally localized to the lateral semicircular canal[11]. Because of its structure, rarely do any otoliths cause BPPV symptoms in the anterior canal. Whereas the anatomical makeup of the individual canals requires both unique diagnostic testing and treatment, we will look at each canal individually.

Posterior Canal

As discussed, the most common location for otolith involvement in BPPV is within the posterior semicircular canal. It is thought that the positioning of the posterior canal allows dislodged otoliths to most easily fall into it first, which is evidenced by the high rate of posterior canal BPPV.

Diagnosis of BPPV in the posterior canal most often uses the Dix-Hallpike positioning test[17]. This test isolates the posterior canal, and therefore any otoliths within the canal are able to move along the length of the canal. It has been suggested to test the left side first as right-side BPPV is more common[17]. Also, both sides should be tested in order to ensure that BPPV is not occurring in both ears.

To conduct the Dix-Hallpike test, the patient is seated at the end of a table, looking 45 degrees to the side, in the same direction as the affected ear (i.e. left ear posterior canal BPPV would require looking left at 45 degrees). Without moving the position of the head, the patient is then quickly laid down, with the head extending over the end of the table so that it is slightly lower than the body. Once the medical professional notices nystagmus – which can take up to 30 seconds to occur – the patient is returned to the beginning position (seated upright). The clinician also asks the patient if he or she is experiencing any symptoms of vertigo or dizziness, or feels as if he or she is falling[55].

In some cases as outlined below, a "half Dix-Hallpike" maneuver can be used to test for the less common cupulolithiasis of the posterior canal, as it is designed to position the affected cupula so as to be fully stimulated by the pull of gravity[17]. For this test, the patient's head is again turned to 45 degrees toward the side being tested, but instead of moving the patient into a supine position, he or she is only brought to the side approximately 60 degrees. Then, the patient's head is turned approximately 180 degrees to the other side, which if effective, instigates a less intense nystagmus that is beating in the opposite direction.

Diagnosis of posterior canal BPPV in response to the Dix-Hallpike test is indicated when there is upward-beating (i.e. 'vertical'), torsional nystagmus that results in the top portion of the patient's eyes beating repeatedly toward the lower ear[11, 28]. Typically, nystagmus begins within two to five seconds and lasts on average 30 seconds, though nystagmus can last up to one minute. Approximately one out of four patients, however, have no nystagmus in response to this test[28]. Once the 30 seconds has passed, the patient is returned to a seated position, which often results in the nystagmus reversing direction[56]. If the Dix-Hallpike test is repeated again, the nystagmus is typically lessened in what is known as 'fatigability'[11, 56].

The Barany society released a consensus document put out by the Committee for the Classification of Vestibular Disorders in 2015. In this document, they outlined several diagnostic criteria relating to BPPV in the posterior canal. For canalolithiasis of the posterior canal, four criteria should be met for an official diagnosis. These conditions are[14]:

A. Recurrent attacks of BPPV or positional dizziness, provoked by lying down or turning over in the supine (i.e. lying on one's back) position
B. Duration of attacks of less than one minute
C. Positional nystagmus that is elicited after a latency of one second to a few seconds by the Dix-Hallpike maneuver or Semont maneuver.
    a. The nystagmus is a combination of torsional nystagmus with the 'upper pole' of the eyes beating toward the lower ear combined with vertical nystagmus beating upward (toward the forehead, typically lasting less than one minute)
D. Not attributable to another disorder

Cupulolithiasis of the posterior canal is also a possible cause of BPPV. For this condition, the Barany society has outlined the following diagnostic criteria:

A. Recurrent attacks of BPPV or positional dizziness triggered by lying down or turning over in the supine position
B. Positional nystagmus elicited after brief latency (or no latency) by a half Dix-Hallpike maneuver, with the eyes beating torsionally toward the lower ear, and lasting greater than one minute
C. Not attributable to another disorder

Horizontal semicircular canal

Otolith involvement within the horizontal canal occurs less often than the posterior canal, but is still highly treatable. For the horizontal canal, patients are diagnosed via the head-roll / log-roll test. Here, the patient lies on his or her back and the head is turned 90 degrees to the left and to the right. Horizontal semicircular canal involvement is diagnosed when nystagmus occurs in either direction, and regardless of the position, the eyes will exhibit nystagmus by beating either toward the ground (geotropic nystagmus) or ceiling (apogeotropic nystagmus).

Because either direction of head movement can induce nystagmus with horizontal canal involvement, the affected ear is usually diagnosed by determining which direction of head movement induces the more powerful nystagmus. When that direction is determined, the eyes will be beating towards the affected ear[28].

Specific to canalolithiasis of the horizontal canal, the Barany society has outlined four diagnostic criteria[14]:

A. Recurrent attacks of positional vertigo or positional dizziness provoked by lying down or turning over in the supine position
B. Duration of attacks of less than one minute
C. Positional nystagmus elicited after a brief latency or no latency by the supine roll test, with eyes beating horizontally toward the undermost ear with the head turned to either side and lasting less than one minute
D. Not attributable to another disorder

Cupulolithiasis of the horizontal canal has its own set of diagnostic criteria, which have been outlined as[14]:

A. Recurrent attacks of BPPV or positional dizziness provoked by lying down or turning over in the supine position
B. Positional nystagmus elicited after a brief latency or no latency by the supine roll test, beating horizontally toward the uppermost ear with the head turned to either side (apogeotropic direction-changing nystagmus), and lasting greater than one minute
C. Not attributable to any other disorder

To test for horizontal canal BPPV, two predominant tests are used, the supine roll – also known as the Pagnini-McClure test – and the bow and lean test. We will discuss each of these tests next.

Supine Roll, or Pagnini-McClure test

To perform the supine roll test, the patient lies prone (on his or her stomach) with their head over the end of a table, flexed forward approximately 30 degrees. Then, either the patient or the examiner moves the head back and forth while the examiner looks for evidence of nystagmus and vertigo.

Bow and lean test

The bow and lean test is recommended to be used after the supine roll test has been performed[55]. Here, the patient either leans forward approximately 60 degrees, or backwards approximately 30 degrees. If experiencing canalolithiasis, leaning forward is expected to cause nystagmus that beats toward the affected ear[55] while the backwards lean should cause nystagmus that beats toward the opposite ear. Conversely, a patient experiencing cupulolithiasis would experience nystagmus occurring in the opposite direction as occurs with canalolithiasis.

Anterior semicircular canal

Though rare, it is possible that otoliths can enter the anterior canal and trigger the effects of BPPV. Because of the structure and location of the anterior semicircular canal, it is difficult for otoliths to enter the canal unless the head is upside down, as otoliths entering the canal during a normal upright head position would require the otoliths to move against gravity to enter either end of the canal. As such, the frequency of anterior canal BPPV occurs with much less frequency compared to posterior or horizontal canal BPPV.

Diagnosis for anterior canal canalolithiasis is made by using the Dix-Hallpike test which produces a downward-beating nystagmus that lasts less than a minute[10]. Patients will also exhibit a torsional nystagmus that is clockwise for an affected left ear, and counterclockwise when the right ear is affected. Patients suspected of anterior semicircular canal BPPV are recommended to be evaluated for central nervous system (i.e. brain) lesions, although central lesions are rarely found[28]. The Barany society has outlined diagnostic criteria for canalolithiasis of the anterior canal as follows:

A. Recurrent attacks of BPPV or positional dizziness provoked by lying down or turning over in the supine position
B. Attacks having a duration of less than one minute
C. Positional nystagmus elicited either immediately or after a latency of one or a few seconds by the Dix-Hallpike maneuver (in one or both ears) or in the supine straight head-hanging position, beating predominantly vertically downward, and lasting less than one minute
D. Not attributable to another disorder.

Treatment of BPPV

As outlined in an earlier chapter, BPPV often resolves itself without the need for treatment. When BPPV does not resolve spontaneously, treatment can be performed which utilizes specific body movements to reposition the otoliths back into the saccule and utricle. In fact, the success of the repositioning maneuvers has generally limited surgical intervention to only those BPPV cases which become intractable in nature. Much like diagnosing BPPV, treatment is dependent upon which semicircular canals are affected.

Please note – images were purposely not included with the maneuvers outlined in this chapter. All procedures discussed next should first be performed under the supervision of a medical professional trained in canalith repositioning, and all repositioning should be performed only after an actual diagnosis of BPPV by a medical professional trained in the various types of BPPV. As such, the following information in this chapter is provided for informational purposes only, in order to outline the various repositioning techniques commonly used to remove otoliths from the semicircular canals. These techniques should not be performed at home unless directed by a vestibular-trained medical professional.

Posterior Semicircular Canal

Two main repositioning maneuvers are used in treating posterior canal BPPV – the Epley maneuver and the Sermont procedure. The Epley maneuver has undergone a series of modifications over the years, starting initially with the use of a vibrating device held against the jaw to help facilitate movement of the otoliths within the ear and requiring an upright head posture for one or more days after the procedure. More recently, the use of the vibrating device has become relatively rare as it has been reported that use of a vibrating device has no effect on the outcome of the procedure[57]. Furthermore, upright head position has largely been discontinued as research has found no improved benefits in doing so[58, 59]. As a result of these findings, the procedure has been renamed the modified Epley maneuver.

Modified Epley Maneuver

Treatment of posterior canal BPPV is most successfully accomplished with the modified Epley maneuver[55]. Performing the Epley maneuver involves starting with the patient sitting upright. Assuming that the patient's right-side posterior canal is affected, the patient's head is turned to 45 degrees to the right, after which he or she is moved backwards to a lying-down position with the head hanging back over the table, slightly downward (at approximately 30 degrees of neck extension) and still turned at a 45-degree angle. At this point, nystagmus is expected to occur, and treatment is paused until the nystagmus stops. The patient's head is then rotated 90 degrees so that he or she is now looking over the opposite shoulder as occurred during the starting position. Then, with the patient's head staying in the same position (45 degrees), the patient is rolled onto his or her left side, which will now place the head in a position so that the patient is looking down at the floor. This position is then maintained until any evident nystagmus ceases. Finally, the patient sits up while the head remains looking down at the floor.

Modified Sermont, or "Liberatory" Maneuver

Not as well studied as the Epley maneuver, the Sermont maneuver has been shown effective at treating posterior canal BPPV. One study found that 87% of patients had no vertigo 24 hours after the procedure[60]. Though not well researched, evidence suggests that the Sermont maneuver is not as effective as the Epley maneuver for treating posterior canal BPPV[61].

To perform the test, the patient is seated on a table. Assuming right semicircular canal involvement, the patient will turn his or her head to the left at a 45-degree angle. The patient is then quickly brought down to a lying position on their right side by the examiner, and this position is held for one minute. Very quickly, the patient is moved from their right side up and over to their left side in no more than 1.5 seconds, which now puts their maintained head position as looking down at the ground. By moving quickly, centrifugal force is generated within the canal that can help facilitate movement of the otoliths. After holding the downward-facing position for one minute, the patient is returned to a seated position.

Brandt-Daroff Exercises/Maneuver

Though not a repositioning treatment, Brandt-Daroff exercises actually paved the way for the Sermont maneuver. Brandt-Daroff exercises mimic the Sermont maneuver, but are performed much slower and can typically be completed without the assistance of a second person.

To perform a repetition of the Brandt-Daroff maneuver, a patient sits upright with the knees bent, allowing the feet to drop down over the end of a table or bed. Assuming BPPV within the right ear, the patient turns his or her head to the left approximately 45 degrees. Next, the patient lies down on their right side for 30 seconds so that their affected ear is against the table or bed. The patient then sits upright again for 30 seconds. Next, the patient turns his or her head 45 degrees to the left and lays over to their left side for 30 seconds before again returning to a seated position.

Studies consistently find that the Epley maneuver is more effective at eliminating BPPV symptoms than the Brandt-Daroff exercises[62, 63]. However, it must be understood that the Brandt-Daroff is not a repositioning treatment but rather a set of exercises that was later modified into the Sermont maneuver.

Half-somersault / Foster Maneuver

Similar to the Brandt-Daroff maneuver, the half-somersault was developed in 2012 by a BPPV sufferer as an exercise rather than a specific maneuver. The half-somersault exercises were designed such that patients could perform the exercises at home without an assistant[64].

To perform the half-somersault procedure, patients first kneel on the floor and then sit back so that their buttocks are resting against their heels. The following steps are then conducted assuming a right-side posterior canal BPPV, with each step being held for approximately 15 seconds. The procedure begins by having the patient quickly look up toward an area of the ceiling that is directly above them. Next, the patient should lean forward, placing the top of the head on the floor and tucking the chin in against the knees. Next, the head is turned 45 degrees to the right. While maintaining the same 45-degrees of head position, the patient then raises their torso up until the elbows are straight (similar to performing a push-up), resulting in the head, shoulders, and back all being at approximately the same level. Finally, the head is fully raised while maintaining the same 45 degree angle.

Horizontal (Lateral) Semicircular Canal

Horizontal canal movement of otoliths can occur through several treatment options. Which way the patient should roll is largely dependent upon recognition of the affected ear. Unlike the posterior canal, nystagmus in the horizontal canal can appear similar on the left and the right side, making it difficult to discern which ear is affected. It has been recommended that the examiner modify repositioning maneuvers as necessary to account for the difficulty in localizing the affected ear as well as the location of the otoliths[55].

Barbecue Roll, Lempert Maneuver

Once the affected ear has been determined, a patient performing a BBQ roll lies on his or her back with their head raised approximately 30 degrees above the table. Next, the head is rotated 90 degrees toward the affected side and held for either 30 seconds or until any elicited nystagmus concludes. The patient's head is then rotated back to neutral and then 90 degrees toward the opposite side for 30 seconds, followed by having the patient roll over into a prone (stomach-down), position for 30 seconds. The patient is then rotated 90 degrees onto the affected side again which places their affected ear in the down position. Finally, the patient returns to a seated position.

Gufoni Maneuver

For the Gufoni maneuver, the patient starts in a seated position. Next, the patient remains in a head-neutral position and lies down quickly to their side for two minutes – toward the patient's affected side if apogeotropic nystagmus is present, and their unaffected side if the nystagmus is geotropic in nature. Next, the patient moves his or her head 45 degrees up or down for an additional two minutes, dependent upon the type of nystagmus present. His or her head should move up 45 degrees for two minutes if apogeotropic nystagmus is present and down 45 degrees if the nystagmus is geotropic in nature.

Anterior Canal

As stated earlier, BPPV resulting from otoliths in the anterior canal is the rarest form, largely due to the fact that the position of the anterior canal makes it difficult for otoliths to enter the anterior canal unless the head is positioned upside-down. Furthermore, even in the event of cupulolithiasis of the anterior canal, the constant pull of gravity during upright-head positioning can result in removal of any otoliths from the canal[55]. Nevertheless, anterior canal BPPV cases have been reported, and there is a relatively successful maneuver for removing the otoliths from the canal.

One therapeutic treatment has become the most popular for canalolithiasis of the anterior canal, and may be the simplest[10]. Here, the patient starts in a seated position, then is quickly laid back with his or her head hanging off the end of the table such that the top of the head is pointing down. Next, the patient's head is raised as if to look down at his or her feet, followed by a return to the seated position.

Summary

Treatment of BPPV has been shown to be quite successful through the use of relatively simple repositioning procedures that take advantage of the design of the semicircular canals in conjunction with gravity to move the otoliths back into the utricle and saccule area. As noted earlier, it is important that an individual is first evaluated by a medical professional before performing repositioning procedures so as to ensure that the proper repositioning technique is utilized. Otherwise, even with classic types of BPPV, incorrect repositioning maneuvers will have no effect in moving the otoliths out of the canal.

Chapter 6: Ear conditions similar to BPPV

OF ALL THE CONDITIONS of the ear that can trigger vertigo and/or balance issues, BPPV should be considered one of the more minor types. While the bouts of vertigo associated with certain head movements can be inopportune at times, such as when reaching up toward a shelf or while taking a shower, the actual cause of the vertigo associated with BPPV is believed to be due to small otoliths causing the nerves of the inner ear to fire inadvertently. When the head is not in a particular position, there is no effect on the nerve and the vestibular system functions as normal. Other vertigo-triggering conditions of the inner ear are not as harmless as BPPV, and it is important to differentiate these other medical conditions from BPPV. Therefore, this chapter serves to outline conditions of the ear capable of inducing vertigo, along with common signs and/or symptoms of each condition.

Patients suffering from vertigo and/or dizziness should understand that they are not alone, as over one-third of Americans will seek medical care for dizziness in their lifetime[65]. However, it is important to point out that both dizziness and vertigo are merely symptoms, and medical practitioners will first look for the underlying cause of each rather than treating the actual symptom. In some cases, vertigo can be due to a condition as minor as an allergy that induces ear congestion. Other times, it can be more involved such as being due to a type of neuritis. Despite the array of potential causes of vertigo, this chapter will focus on those conditions which are similar to BPPV in that they trigger dizziness and/or vertigo as the result of inner ear maladies.

Allergies / Congestion

All of us have likely experienced a head cold or an allergy attack that affects our inner ear and causes dizziness. Dizziness related to either a cold or allergy issue is relatively harmless, and usually passes within a few days. In many cases, the dizziness results not from a problem within the labyrinth system but rather an inability of the

Eustachian tube – a passageway designed to drain excess fluid from our middle ear to our throat – to properly remove excess fluid or mucus from the middle ear. Proper diagnosis of ear congestion should be made by a medical professional, and if that is indeed the case, medication can often help reduce the associated symptoms.

Labyrinthitis

Inflammation of the inner ear – whether from a virus or bacteria – can lead to labyrinthitis. Typically, viral labyrinthitis affects older individuals (e.g. over 30 years of age), which separates labyrinthitis from the more common, simple ear infections that children often incur. In many cases, viral or bacterial labyrinthitis lasts no more than two or three weeks, though more severe cases can last longer and require significant intervention.

Many cases of viral labyrinthitis are thought to result from a simple head or chest cold that spreads to the inner ear. Treatment of viral meningitis is usually performed symptomatically, while bacterial labyrinthitis can be treated using a prescription of antibiotics.

Ménière's Disease

Ménière's disorder is a condition thought to result from problems with the fluid regulation system of the inner ear. Ménière's patients typically experience an ongoing degree of unsteadiness and ear pressure or fullness intermixed with bouts of acute vertigo, nausea, and vomiting that can last several hours.

Several underlying causes of Ménière's have been proposed, including water regulation, endolymph reabsorption anomalies, vascular abnormalities, and autoimmune factors[66, 67]. Fluid regulation in the middle ear is thought to be one of the main triggers of Ménière's. For example, water channels, which regulate the transport of water across membranes, have been implicated as a possible cause of Ménière's[68, 69]. Unexpected reductions or increases in the number of water channels can influence the balance of fluid on each side of a membrane.

Similarly, some researchers suggest that Ménière's patients have a diminished capacity to regulate fluid within their inner ear[70]. Consequently, fluctuations in the inner ear fluid are not well tolerated in Ménière's patients. This is thought to lead to fluid imbalances that contribute to many of the symptoms encountered by Ménière's patients. Electrolytes such as sodium that are known to play a role in the body's fluid regulation are commonly restricted in Ménière's patients in order to reduce potential fluctuations within the middle ear.

Other potential underlying causes of Ménière's disease include autoimmune disorders[71], the herpes virus[72], cervical disorders[73] and stress[74]. Whereas no definitive underlying source of Ménière's has been discovered, it is vital that research continue to investigate these and all logical possibilities.

Due in large part to the complexity and sensitivity of the vestibular system, Ménière's remains a complicated disease. During acute attacks Ménière's can be extremely debilitating, followed by months or years of the same individual reporting almost no symptoms. At present there remains no cure for Ménière's, though symptoms can often be controlled through lifestyle modifications including strict monitoring of sodium intake. Medication can also be helpful in controlling the symptoms of Ménière's.

Vestibular Neuritis

Vestibular neuritis is associated with vertigo, nausea, vomiting, and imbalance and is thought to be due to viral inflammation of the vestibular nerve[75]. The condition is acute in nature with symptoms lasting from a few days to several weeks, but up to half of those suffering from vestibular neuritis can experience symptoms much longer[11, 76]. Vestibular neuritis has been reported to account for nearly 10% of all dizziness-related medical visits[39]. Interestingly, viral epidemics trigger an increased incidence of vestibular neuritis, lending evidence to its likely inflammatory origins.

Patients exhibiting vestibular neuritis will present with acute, severe vertigo[77]. The most severe portion of the attack can last for one to two days and then gradually subside over the following weeks. Motion may worsen the vertigo, and some patients experience nausea and vomiting in conjunction with the vertigo[77]. Additional symptoms include nystagmus as well as a walking pattern in which the patient tends to lean toward the affected ear's side.

Treatment of vestibular neuritis includes symptomatic care along with vestibular rehabilitation, which can begin as soon as tolerable after cessation of immediate symptoms[77]. Vestibular rehabilitation has been reported to be successful for neuritis patients when compared against patients receiving no therapy[78]. If vestibular neuritis is severe, short-term hospitalization may be required[77].

Vestibular Migraine

Vestibular migraines are among the more common vestibular disorders, affecting up to 1% of the population[79, 80] and up to 11% of patients seeking treatment in dizziness-related clinics[81]. Vestibular migraines are also relatively common in children, having been reported to occur in nearly 3% of children aged 6-12 years of age[82]. Like Ménière's disease, vestibular migraine has no universally accepted definition which can in turn limit recognition of vestibular migraines in affected patients. Only recently were the diagnostic criteria established which include the following[81].

1. Vestibular migraine

   A. At least 5 episodes with vestibular symptoms of moderate or severe intensity, lasting 5 minutes to 72 hours

   B. Current or previous history of migraine with or without aura according to the

International Classification of Headache Disorders (ICHD)

C. One or more migraine features with at least 50% of the vestibular episodes:

– headache with at least two of the following characteristics: one sided location, pulsating quality, moderate or severe pain intensity, aggravation by routine physical activity

– photophobia and phonophobia

– visual aura

D. Not better accounted for by another vestibular or ICHD diagnosis

2. Probable vestibular migraine

A. At least 5 episodes with vestibular symptoms of moderate or severe intensity, lasting 5 min to 72 hours

B. Only one of the criteria B and C for vestibular migraine is fulfilled (migraine history or migraine features during the episode)

C. Not better accounted for by another vestibular or ICHD diagnosis

The predominant symptoms of vestibular migraine include vertigo in combination with headache, and these two symptoms often occur relatively close to each other[77]. Other symptoms can include transient hearing fluctuations[83], nausea, vomiting, and a sensitivity to motion sickness[81]. Some patients have reported triggering of their migraine in response to dehydration, lack of sleep, or certain foods, but the relationship between these characteristics and vestibular migraines has not been well-studied[81]. Evidence of effective treatment of vestibular migraines is limited. Patients who respond favorably to anti-migraine medication have occurred, but the evidence is lacking as to overall effectiveness[84].

Chapter 7: BPPV and Quality of Life

WHILE THE INITIAL effects of BPPV can be quite frightening, most patients live relatively normal lives. This lies in part due to the 'positional' component of BPPV in that the effects are not always present but rather are dependent upon the position of the head. Avoiding those positions which induce the effects of BPPV allow for minimal if any interruption. However, some individuals may be more impacted by the effects of BPPV as a result of their occupation requiring them to be in positions that may trigger the symptoms. For example, painters or mechanics are often required to look upwards or be in a supine position which can trigger the effects of BPPV. Such individuals often learn unique ways to avoid the triggering positions, thereby allowing them to avoid the symptoms of BPPV.

Unlike many other ear-related conditions, BPPV is not associated with hearing loss. Because

BPPV is often activated when a patient is lying down, sleep can be problematic unless adjustments are made. It is not uncommon for individuals to avoid lying down flat in bed as is traditionally done, with some patients preferring to sleep in a semi-reclined or semi-sitting position[17]. Furthermore, patients will often avoid turning over while lying down[17].

Patients with BPPV are more likely to have depression[7]. This brings with it reduced quality of life scores among BPPV patients. Furthermore, BPPV patients are more likely to have sustained a fall within the prior three months[30]. Within the geriatric population, BPPV increases the risk of falls[85], a particularly problematic consequence given the higher risk of osteoporosis, fractures, or injury within the older population[85, 86]. This, coupled with the fact that patients older than 70 take longer to seek help for their BPPV make the geriatric population a particular concern for managing BPPV[87]. Individuals with BPPV are more likely to report a reduced quality of life[88]. Seventy percent of BPPV sufferers engage in 'avoidance behaviors' which means that they purposely avoid certain actions that can trigger BPPV[89]. For example, they may avoid sleeping on their back, or looking upwards. And because of BPPV and its effects on balance, patients with BPPV are more likely to have suffered a fall within the past three months[30].

Not only does BPPV affect quality of life, it can also have a financial impact[90]. The costs for caring for BPPV exceed $2,000 per patient in year 2000 dollars[91], equivalent to approximately $2,900 for treatment of BPPV in 2018. However, much of this cost was suspected to be from unnecessary diagnostic measures and ineffective therapy, likely due to the fact that BPPV has a low rate of recognition among primary care physicians[54]. Hopefully, more focused diagnosis as well as a better understanding of the disease will help alleviate costs.

Particularly interesting about BPPV is that one study found that all measures relating to quality of life improved after canalith repositioning[88]. Furthermore, social function and mental health scores improved significantly, indicating that these two measures exhibited the most improvement after canalith repositioning. In addition, the Dizziness Handicap Inventory (short form) survey responses indicated that vertigo decreased significantly after canalith repositioning.

Because an older population is more likely to suffer from BPPV, it is important to understand how the disease affects this population as well. Researchers have found that canalith repositioning can significantly improve scores relating to body pain, vitality, social function, and mental health.

Chapter 8: In Conclusion

As this book has outlined, BPPV can be both a highly involved as well as highly variable condition. As a former sufferer of BPPV, the overwhelming initial symptoms associated with BPPV, combined with the uncertainty of the condition are largely what pushed me towards writing this book. I did not have a good resource during my time living with BPPV, and I hope that this book has served as an effective resource for you as you live with or recover from BPPV.

Describing vertigo to someone who has never had it – especially vertigo that only occurs in response to certain head positions – can be difficult in comparison to something like a head cold or a sore shoulder, both conditions from which pretty much everyone has suffered. In writing this book I felt that by detailing the events occurring with BPPV as well as describing my own experiences, BPPV sufferers could not only better understand their condition but also help others understand the condition as well. And, when faced with the inevitable questions from friends and family such as "BP-what???", the information in this book will hopefully provide you a solid foundation for outlining the basics of just what is occurring inside of the ear when BPPV hits.

Regardless of how you use the information, I hope that this book has been informative for you. In writing it, I have learned a great deal more about BPPV than I knew previously, and I encourage you to also continue to expand your knowledge of this condition. Even though our techniques in treating BPPV has progressed immensely in the past 25 years, as BPPV research continues to expand, further advanced therapies and treatments are likely to follow close behind. As medical professionals begin to integrate these advancements into clinical practice, it is hoped that treatments become even more effective, and possibly even simpler to perform.

If you currently have BPPV, whether traditional or intractable in nature, continue to work carefully with your physician and follow the directions given so as to ensure the best possible treatment outcomes. Be mindful of the potential for recurrent episodes of BPPV, and always be wary of potential scams relating to treatments and devices. And if your BPPV relief is not quick, look for support methods including online groups as well as that support which you can find through building a strong social network. BPPV can be a highly disruptive condition, and those around you need to be aware of your situation, your frustrations, and your difficulties in order to assist you in the best possible care. As you may have already learned, sometimes just lending an understanding ear can make a world of difference.

In closing, I wish you the best of luck in your treatment and journey with BPPV. I have been there, and I myself like many others have had a successful outcome. Not everyone will be 100% cured, but know that current medical techniques are being refined and researched to help improve our treatment of BPPV.

Glossary

Ampulla: an expanded area of the semicircular canals that houses the cupula

Anterior canal: one of the semicircular canals that is responsible for detecting motion of the head such as occurs when nodding one's head to indicate "yes"

Apogeotropic: a type of nystagmus in which the eyes beat repeatedly toward the ceiling

Benign: not harmful

Canalith: see "otolith"

Canalithiasis: a type of BPPV thought to be triggered by free-floating otoliths within the semicircular canal that, when the head is positioned at a certain angle, disrupt fluid flow within the canal and trigger the effects of BPPV

Canalith repositioning / "Epley Maneuver": a series of positions that a BPPV patient is placed in with the intent of causing otoliths within the affected ear to be moved back to the utricle

Cochlea: the organ of the inner ear shaped like a snail's shell which is responsible for receiving vibrations from the eardrum and converting them into electrical signals for transmission to the brain

Compound: a substance made up of two or more individual elements

Cupula: a structure within the semicircular canals that detects movement of endolymph in order to allow the brain to detect head motion

Cupulolithiasis: a type of BPPV thought to be triggered when otoliths of the inner ear adhere to the cupula of the inner ear

Dizziness: a sensation that results in the patient feeling as if he or she is spinning or moving while remaining stationary

Endolymph: the potassium-rich fluid contained within the membranous labyrinth of the ear

Equilibrium: a state of overall balance

Geotropic: nystagmus in which the eyes beat repeatedly toward the ground

Hair Cell: sensory receptors located within the auditory and vestibular organs of the ear that transmit a signal to the brain in response to detection of head movement or sound vibrations

Horizontal canal: one of the semicircular canals that is responsible for detecting motion of the head such as occurs when shaking one's head to indicate "no"

Inner Ear: the portion of the ear within the temporal bone that contains the semicircular canals and cochlea

Intractable BPPV: a type of BPPV which has either not responded to multiple canalith repositioning attempts, or continues to recur despite successful repositioning attempts

Latent nystagmus: a type of nystagmus that occurs when covering one eye, which then beats toward the uncovered eye

Ménière's Disease: a condition of the inner ear comprised of symptoms that include vertigo, tinnitus, hearing loss, and the sensation of ear fullness

Middle Ear: the central cavity of the inner ear comprised of the empty space within the temporal bone located inside of the eardrum

Nystagmus: involuntary eye movement

Organ of Corti: an organ of the inner ear that is responsible for transmitting sound vibrations into nerve signals

Otolith: small calcium-based structures of the inner ear designed to assist with detecting head motion

Otolithic Membrane: the gelatinous portion of the inner ear that is embedded with otoliths and serves as a material that the ear can use to aid in the detection of head motion

Outer Ear: That portion of the ear that is visible, along with the auditory canal

Paroxysmal: sudden onset

Posterior canal: one of the semicircular canals that is responsible for detecting motion of the head such as occurs when placing an ear on its same-side shoulder

Prone: Lying face-down

Rotatory nystagmus: a type of nystagmus in which the top of the eye rotates toward the ear affected with BPPV

Saccule: like the utricle, an area concentrated with sensory nerves with the inner ear and responsible for detecting head movement

Semicircular Canals: three fluid-filled tubes of the inner ear responsible for detecting head movement

Supine: Lying on one's back

Temporal bone: A bone that is positioned at the side and base of the skull which houses the vestibular and hearing organs

Torsional nystagmus: movement of the eye along it's anterior-to-posterior axis

Utricle: like the saccule, an area concentrated with sensory nerves with the inner ear and responsible for detecting head movement

Vertigo: a sensation of spinning that is usually accompanied by a sudden loss of balance

Vestibular nerve: the eighth cranial nerve, responsible for transmitting hearing and sensory information from the inner ear to the brain

References

1. Ekdale, E.G., *Form and function of the mammalian inner ear.* Journal of anatomy, 2016. **228**(2): p. 324-337.
2. Gordon, C.R., et al., *Traumatic benign paroxysmal positional vertigo: diagnosis and treatment.* Harefuah, 2002. **141**(11): p. 944-7, 1012, 1011.
3. Rask-Andersen, H., et al., *Human cochlea: anatomical characteristics and their relevance for cochlear implantation.* The Anatomical Record, 2012. **295**(11): p. 1791-1811.
4. Hudspeth, A., *The hair cells of the inner ear.* Scientific American, 1983. **248**(1): p. 54-65.
5. Walther, L.E., et al., *Detection of human utricular otoconia degeneration in vital specimen and implications for benign paroxysmal positional vertigo.* European Archives of Oto-Rhino-Laryngology, 2014. **271**(12): p. 3133-3138.
6. Andrade, L.R., et al., *Immunogold TEM of otoconin 90 and otolin–relevance to mineralization of otoconia, and pathogenesis of benign positional vertigo.* Hearing research, 2012. **292**(1-2): p. 14-25.

7. Parham, K., *Benign paroxysmal positional vertigo: an integrated perspective.* Advances in otolaryngology, 2014. **2014**.
8. Giacomini, P.G., et al., *Recurrent paroxysmal positional vertigo related to oral contraceptive treatment.* Gynecological endocrinology, 2006. **22**(1): p. 5-8.
9. Schuknecht, H. and R. Ruby, *Cupulolithiasis*, in *Otophysiology*. 1973, Karger Publishers. p. 434-443.
10. Pérez-Vázquez, P. and V. Franco-Gutiérrez, *Treatment of benign paroxysmal positional vertigo. A clinical review.* 收藏, 2017. **4**: p. 002.
11. Bergenius, J., Z. Qing, and D. Maoli, *Benign paroxysmal positional vertigo.* Journal of Otology, 2014. **9**(1): p. 1-6.
12. Bhattacharyya, N., et al., *Clinical practice guideline: Benign paroxysmal positional vertigo (update) executive summary.* Otolaryngology–Head and Neck Surgery, 2017. **156**(3): p. 403-416.
13. Bisdorff, A.R., J.P. Staab, and D.E. Newman-Toker, *Overview of the international classification of vestibular disorders.* Neurologic clinics, 2015. **33**(3): p. 541-550.
14. Von Brevern, M., et al., *Benign paroxysmal positional vertigo: diagnostic criteria.* Journal of Vestibular Research, 2015. **25**(3, 4): p. 105-117.

15. Shim, D.B., et al., *Natural history of horizontal canal benign paroxysmal positional vertigo is truly short.* Journal of neurology, 2015. **262**(1): p. 74-80.
16. Zamergrad, M., et al., *Common Causes of Vertigo and Dizziness in Different Age Groups of Patients.* BioNanoScience, 2017. **7**(2): p. 259-262.
17. Nuti, D., M. Masini, and M. Mandalà, *Benign paroxysmal positional vertigo and its variants*, in *Handbook of clinical neurology*. 2016, Elsevier. p. 241-256.
18. Cambi, J., et al., *Natural course of positional down-beating nystagmus of peripheral origin.* Journal of neurology, 2013. **260**(6): p. 1489-1496.
19. Hornibrook, J., *Benign paroxysmal positional vertigo (BPPV): history, pathophysiology, office treatment and future directions.* International journal of otolaryngology, 2011. **2011**.
20. Simhadri, S., N. Panda, and M. Raghunathan, *Efficacy of particle repositioning maneuver in BPPV: a prospective study.* American journal of otolaryngology, 2003. **24**(6): p. 355-360.
21. Parnes, L.S. and J.A. Mcclure, *Free-floating endolymph particles: a new operative finding during posterior semicircular canal occlusion.* The Laryngoscope, 1992. **102**(9): p. 988-992.

22. Caruso, G. and D. Nuti, *Epidemiological data from 2270 PPV patients.* Audiological medicine, 2005. **3**(1): p. 7-11.
23. Hanley, K., T. O'Dowd, and N. Considine, *A systematic review of vertigo in primary care.* Br J Gen Pract, 2001. **51**(469): p. 666-671.
24. Gizzi, M., S. Ayyagari, and V. Khattar, *The familial incidence of benign paroxysmal positional vertigo.* Acta oto-laryngologica, 1998. **118**(6): p. 774-777.
25. Gross, E.M., et al., *Intractable benign paroxysmal positional vertigo in patients with Meniere's disease.* The Laryngoscope, 2000. **110**(4): p. 655-659.
26. Neuhauser, H., *The epidemiology of dizziness and vertigo,* in *Handbook of clinical neurology*. 2016, Elsevier. p. 67-82.
27. Von Brevern, M., et al., *Epidemiology of benign paroxysmal positional vertigo: a population based study.* Journal of Neurology, Neurosurgery & Psychiatry, 2007. **78**(7): p. 710-715.
28. Kim, J.-S. and D.S. Zee, *Benign paroxysmal positional vertigo.* New England Journal of Medicine, 2014. **370**(12): p. 1138-1147.
29. Kerrigan, M.A., et al., *Prevalence of benign paroxysmal positional vertigo in the young adult population.* PM&R, 2013. **5**(9): p. 778-785.

30. Oghalai, J.S., et al., *Unrecognized benign paroxysmal positional vertigo in elderly patients.* Otolaryngology—Head and Neck Surgery, 2000. **122**(5): p. 630-634.
31. Nunez, R.A., S.P. Cass, and J.M. Furman, *Short-and long-term outcomes of canalith repositioning for benign paroxysmal positional vertigo.* Otolaryngology—Head and Neck Surgery, 2000. **122**(5): p. 647-652.
32. Gordon, C.R., et al., *Is posttraumatic benign paroxysmal positional vertigo different from the idiopathic form?* Archives of Neurology, 2004. **61**(10): p. 1590-1593.
33. Kansu, L., et al., *Long-term follow-up of patients with posterior canal benign paroxysmal positional vertigo.* Acta oto-laryngologica, 2010. **130**(9): p. 1009-1012.
34. Soto-Varela, A., et al., *Are the three canals equally susceptible to benign paroxysmal positional vertigo?* Audiology and Neurotology, 2013. **18**(5): p. 327-334.
35. Vibert, D., M. Kompis, and R. Häusler, *Benign paroxysmal positional vertigo in older women may be related to osteoporosis and osteopenia.* Annals of Otology, Rhinology & Laryngology, 2003. **112**(10): p. 885-889.

36. Büki, B., et al., *Vitamin D deficiency and benign paroxysmal positioning vertigo.* Medical hypotheses, 2013. **80**(2): p. 201-204.
37. Imai, T., et al., *Natural course of the remission of vertigo in patients with benign paroxysmal positional vertigo.* Neurology, 2005. **64**(5): p. 920-921.
38. Burton, M.J., T.L. Eby, and R.M. Rosenfeld, *Extracts from the Cochrane library: modifications of the Epley (canalith repositioning) maneuver for posterior canal benign paroxysmal positional vertigo.* Otolaryngology--Head and Neck Surgery, 2012. **147**(3): p. 407-411.
39. Neuhauser, H.K. and T. Lempert. *Vertigo: epidemiologic aspects*. in *Seminars in neurology*. 2009. © Thieme Medical Publishers.
40. Von Brevern, M., et al., *Benign paroxysmal positional vertigo predominantly affects the right labyrinth.* Journal of Neurology, Neurosurgery & Psychiatry, 2004. **75**(10): p. 1487-1488.
41. Zucca, G., et al., *Why do benign paroxysmal positional vertigo episodes recover spontaneously?* Journal of Vestibular Research, 1998. **8**(4): p. 325-329.
42. Kveton, J.F. and M. Kashgarian, *Particulate matter within the membranous labyrinth: pathologic or normal?* The American journal of otology, 1994. **15**(2): p. 173-176.

43. Leveque, M., et al., *Surgical therapy in intractable benign paroxysmal positional vertigo.* Otolaryngology—Head and Neck Surgery, 2007. **136**(5): p. 693-698.
44. Choi, S.J., et al., *Clinical features of recurrent or persistent benign paroxysmal positional vertigo.* Otolaryngology--Head and Neck Surgery, 2012. **147**(5): p. 919-924.
45. Parnes, L.S. and R.G. Price-Jones, *Particle repositioning maneuver for benign paroxysmal positional vertigo.* Annals of Otology, Rhinology & Laryngology, 1993. **102**(5): p. 325-331.
46. Horii, A., et al., *Intractable benign paroxysmal positioning vertigo: long-term follow-up and inner ear abnormality detected by three-dimensional magnetic resonance imaging.* Otology & Neurotology, 2010. **31**(2): p. 250-255.
47. Parnes, L.S., S.K. Agrawal, and J. Atlas, *Diagnosis and management of benign paroxysmal positional vertigo (BPPV).* Canadian Medical Association Journal, 2003. **169**(7): p. 681-693.
48. Pérez, P., et al., *A Pilot Study Using Intratympanic Methylprednisolone for Treatment of Persistent Posterior Canal Benign Paroxysmal Positional Vertigo.* Journal of International Advanced Otology, 2016. **12**(3).

49. Kaur, J. and K. Shamanna, *Management of Benign Paroxysmal Positional Vertigo: A Comparative Study between Epleys Manouvre and Betahistine.* The international tinnitus journal, 2017. **21**(1): p. 30-34.
50. Smith, T.L., *Evidence-Based Clinical Practice in Otolaryngology, An Issue of Otolaryngologic Clinics-E-Book*. Vol. 45. 2012: Elsevier Health Sciences.
51. Parnes, L.S. and J.A. McClure, *Posterior semicircular canal occlusion for intractable benign paroxysmal positional vertigo.* Annals of Otology, Rhinology & Laryngology, 1990. **99**(5): p. 330-334.
52. Sataloff, R.T. and A.P. Sclafani, *Sataloff's Comprehensive Textbook of Otolaryngology: Head & Neck Surgery: Facial Plastic and Reconstructive Surgery*. Vol. 3. 2015: JP Medical Ltd.
53. Money, K.E. and J.W. Scott, *Functions of separate sensory receptors of nonauditory labyrinth of the cat.* American Journal of Physiology-Legacy Content, 1962. **202**(6): p. 1211-1220.
54. Hansson, E.E., N.-O. Månsson, and A. Håkansson, *Benign paroxysmal positional vertigo among elderly patients in primary health care.* Gerontology, 2005. **51**(6): p. 386-389.

55. Gold, D.R., et al., *Repositioning maneuvers for benign paroxysmal positional vertigo.* Current treatment options in neurology, 2014. **16**(8): p. 307.
56. Dix, M. and C. Hallpike, *LXXVIII The Pathology, Symptomatology and Diagnosis of Certain Common Disorders of the Vestibular System.* Annals of Otology, Rhinology & Laryngology, 1952. **61**(4): p. 987-1016.
57. Macias, J.D., et al., *Vibration with the canalith repositioning maneuver: a prospective randomized study to determine efficacy.* The Laryngoscope, 2004. **114**(6): p. 1011-1014.
58. Moon, S.J., et al., *The effect of postural restrictions in the treatment of benign paroxysmal positional vertigo.* European Archives of Oto-Rhino-Laryngology and Head & Neck, 2005. **262**(5): p. 408-411.
59. Fyrmpas, G., et al., *Are postural restrictions after an Epley maneuver unnecessary? First results of a controlled study and review of the literature.* Auris Nasus Larynx, 2009. **36**(6): p. 637-643.
60. Mandalà, M., et al., *Double-blind randomized trial on short-term efficacy of the Semont maneuver for the treatment of posterior canal benign paroxysmal positional vertigo.* Journal of neurology, 2012. **259**(5): p. 882-885.

61. Sen, K., A. Sarkar, and A. Raghavan, *Comparative efficacy of epley and semont maneuver in benign paroxysmal positional vertigo: A prospective randomized double-blind study.* Astrocyte, 2016. **3**(2): p. 96.
62. Radtke, A., et al., *A modified Epley's procedure for self-treatment of benign paroxysmal positional vertigo.* Neurology, 1999. **53**(6): p. 1358-1358.
63. Amor-Dorado, J.C., et al., *Particle repositioning maneuver versus Brandt-Daroff exercise for treatment of unilateral idiopathic BPPV of the posterior semicircular canal: a randomized prospective clinical trial with short-and long-term outcome.* Otology & Neurotology, 2012. **33**(8): p. 1401-1407.
64. Foster, C.A., et al., *A comparison of two home exercises for benign positional vertigo: Half somersault versus Epley Maneuver.* Audiology and Neurotology Extra, 2012. **2**(1): p. 16-23.
65. Agrawal, Y., et al., *Disorders of balance and vestibular function in US adults: data from the National Health and Nutrition Examination Survey, 2001-2004.* Archives of internal medicine, 2009. **169**(10): p. 938-944.
66. Minor, L., D. Schessel, and J. Carey, *Meniere's Disease.* Current Opinion in Neurology, 2004. **17**(1): p. 9-16.

67. Baloh, R.W., *Prosper Meniere and his disease.* Archives of neurology, 2001. **58**(7): p. 1151-1156.
68. Ishiyama, G., et al., *Meniere's disease: histopathology, cytochemistry, and imaging.* Annals of the New York Academy of Sciences, 2015. **1343**(1): p. 49-57.
69. Candreia, C., N. Schmuziger, and N. Gürtler, *Molecular analysis of aquaporin genes 1 to 4 in patients with Meniere's disease.* Cellular physiology and biochemistry, 2010. **26**(4-5): p. 787-792.
70. Rauch, S.D., *Clinical hints and precipitating factors in patients suffering from Meniere's disease.* Otolaryngologic Clinics of North America, 2010. **43**(5): p. 1011-1017.
71. Kangasniemi, E. and E. Hietikko, *The theory of autoimmunity in Meniere's disease is lacking evidence.* Auris Nasus Larynx, 2017.
72. Vrabec, J.T., *Herpes simplex virus and Meniere's disease.* The Laryngoscope, 2003. **113**(9): p. 1431-1438.
73. Bjorne, A., A. Berven, and G. Agerberg, *Cervical signs and symptoms in patients with Meniere's disease: a controlled study.* CRANIO®, 1998. **16**(3): p. 194-202.
74. Söderman, A.C.H., et al., *Stress as a Trigger of Attacks in Menière's Disease. A Case-Crossover*

Study. The laryngoscope, 2004. **114**(10): p. 1843-1848.

75. Schuknecht, H.F. and K. Kitamura, *Vestibular neuritis*. Annals of Otology, Rhinology & Laryngology, 1981. **90**(1_suppl): p. 1-19.
76. Perols, J.B., Olle, *Vestibular neuritis: a follow-up study*. Acta oto-laryngologica, 1999. **119**(8): p. 895-899.
77. Wipperman, J., *Dizziness and vertigo*. Primary Care: Clinics in Office Practice, 2014. **41**(1): p. 115-131.
78. Hillier, S.L. and M. McDonnell, *Vestibular rehabilitation for unilateral peripheral vestibular dysfunction*. The Cochrane Library, 2011.
79. Cherchi, M. and T.C. Hain, *Migraine-associated vertigo*. Otolaryngologic Clinics of North America, 2011. **44**(2): p. 367-375.
80. Neuhauser, H., et al., *Migrainous vertigo Prevalence and impact on quality of life*. Neurology, 2006. **67**(6): p. 1028-1033.
81. Lempert, T., et al., *Vestibular migraine: diagnostic criteria*. Journal of Vestibular Research, 2012. **22**(4): p. 167-172.
82. Abu-Arafeh, I. and G. Russell, *Paroxysmal vertigo as a migraine equivalent in children: a population-based study*. Cephalalgia, 1995. **15**(1): p. 22-25.

83. Johnson, G.D., *Medical Management of Migraine-Related Dizziness and Vertigo.* The Laryngoscope, 1998. **108**(S85): p. 1-28.
84. Fotuhi, M., et al., *Vestibular migraine: a critical review of treatment trials.* Journal of neurology, 2009. **256**(5): p. 711-716.
85. Ganança, F.F., et al., *Elderly falls associated with benign paroxysmal positional vertigo.* Brazilian journal of otorhinolaryngology, 2010. **76**(1): p. 113-120.
86. Liao, W.-L., et al., *Benign paroxysmal positional vertigo is associated with an increased risk of fracture: a population-based cohort study.* journal of orthopaedic & sports physical therapy, 2015. **45**(5): p. 406-412.
87. Batuecas-Caletrio, A., et al., *Benign paroxysmal positional vertigo in the elderly.* Gerontology, 2013. **59**(5): p. 408-412.
88. Lopez-Escamez, J., et al., *Classification Committee of the Barany Society; Japan Society for Equilibrium Research; European Academy of Otology and Neurotology (EAONO); Equilibrium Committee of the American Academy of Otolaryngology-Head and Neck Surgery (AAO-HNS); Korean Balance Society. Diagnostic criteria for Menière's disease.* J Vestib Res, 2015. **25**(1): p. 1-7.

89. Von Brevern, M., et al., *Benign paroxysmal positional vertigo: current status of medical management*. Otolaryngology-Head and Neck Surgery, 2004. **130**(3): p. 381-382.
90. Benecke, H., et al., *The burden and impact of vertigo: findings from the REVERT patient registry*. Frontiers in neurology, 2013. **4**: p. 136.
91. Li, J.C., et al., *Cost-effective management of benign positional vertigo using canalith repositioning*. Otolaryngology—Head and Neck Surgery, 2000. **122**(3): p. 334-339.

Image Credits:

Figure 1.1: MedicalArtInc/shutterstock.com
Figure 1.2: Alexilusmedical/shutterstock.com
Figure 1.3: Maxcreatnz/shutterstock.com
Figure 1.4: Designua/shutterstock.com

Other books by Mark Knoblauch

Be sure and check out Mark Knoblauch's other works, including his most recent release, "*Overcoming Meniere's*" which can be found on Amazon.

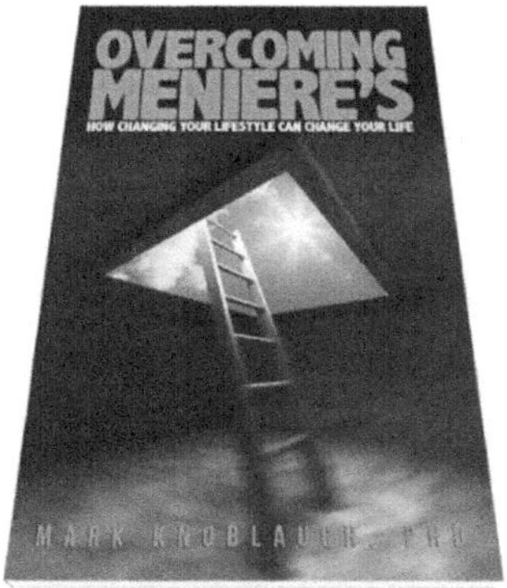

Also be sure to visit www.authorMK.com to learn more about Mark and be first to hear about upcoming book releases. And, sign up for his newsletter to learn about book deals, appearances, and get access to informative videos!

If you felt that what you read in this book was informative, please be sure to post a review on Amazon to let others know.

Made in the USA
Las Vegas, NV
29 October 2026

56836051R00075